Madalina Ilie
Luminita Dascalu
Radu Alexandru Macovei

Helicobacter Pylori Cag A antibodies and their clinical implications

Madalina Ilie
Luminita Dascalu
Radu Alexandru Macovei

Helicobacter Pylori Cag A antibodies and their clinical implications

Correlation of Helicobacter pylori CagA antibodies with treatment resistance, bleeding ulcer and gastric cancer

LAP LAMBERT Academic Publishing

Imprint

Any brand names and product names mentioned in this book are subject to trademark, brand or patent protection and are trademarks or registered trademarks of their respective holders. The use of brand names, product names, common names, trade names, product descriptions etc. even without a particular marking in this work is in no way to be construed to mean that such names may be regarded as unrestricted in respect of trademark and brand protection legislation and could thus be used by anyone.

Cover image: www.ingimage.com

Publisher:
LAP LAMBERT Academic Publishing
is a trademark of
Dodo Books Indian Ocean Ltd. and OmniScriptum S.R.L publishing group

120 High Road, East Finchley, London, N2 9ED, United Kingdom
Str. Armeneasca 28/1, office 1, Chisinau MD-2012, Republic of Moldova, Europe
Managing Directors: Ieva Konstantinova, Victoria Ursu
info@omniscriptum.com

Printed at: see last page
ISBN: 978-3-659-52663-3

HELICOBACTER PYLORI CAG A ANTIBODIES AND THEIR CLINICAL IMPLICATIONS

Correlation of anti-*Helicobacter pylori* CagA-IgG antibodies with resistance to first line treatment, bleeding gastroduodenal ulcers and gastric cancer

Luminita Dascalu, PhD

Assistant Professor of Microbiology, Faculty of Biology- University of Bucharest

Madalina Ilie, MD, PhD

Specialist in internal medicine and gastroenterology, Clinical Emergency Hospital Bucharest; Assistant Professor of Gastroenterology, University of Medicine and Pharmacy Carol Davila

Radu Alexandru Macovei, MD, PhD

Professor of Toxicology, University of Medicine and Pharmacy Carol Davila Bucharest; Head of Department of ICU-Toxicology, Clinical Emergency Hospital Bucharest

Carmen Chifiriuc, Ph D

Professor of Microbiology, Faculty of Biology- University of Bucharest

Gabriel Constantinescu, MD, PhD

Consultant Physician of Gastroenterology, Clinical Emergency Hospital Bucharest; Associate Professor of Gastroenterology, University of Medicine and Pharmacy Carol Davila

Anca Macovei Oprescu, MD, PhD

Specialist in Gastroenterology, Agrippa Ionescu Hospital

Assistant Professor of Gastroenterology, University of Medicine and Pharmacy Carol Davila

Alina Baltac, MD

Fellow in Gastroenterology, Clinical Emergency Hospital Bucharest

Luminita Stanciulescu, MD

Consultant physician and Researcher in Anesthesia and Intesive Care, Clinical Emergency Hospital Bucharest

Contents

1. Introduction

The gastroenterologist Barry Marshall and the pathologist Robin Warren, in the 1980's, fulfilled Koch's postulates for the association between gastritis and the human gastric pathogen *Helicobacter pylori* (Kidd and Modlin, 1998; Warren, 1983; Marshall, 1985). This discovery changed our views of the microbiology and pathology of the human stomach and resulted in Marshall and Warren receiving the 2005 Nobel Prize in Physiology and Medicine.

It has been estimated that half the world's population carries *H. pylori*. Colonization occurs in childhood, persists throughout life and is causing disease mainly in adults (Atherton and Balser, 2009). In most subjects, *H. pylori* is commensal, not related to disease, but the co-evolution of *Homo sapiens* and *H. pylori* throughout millennia may be coming to an end, especially in affluent societies in which marked improvements in home and food sanitation have taken place and antibiotics may be abused to treat minor or to "prevent" infections (Yamaoka et al., 2008). Most infected people remain asymptomatic during their lifetime, and only about 15% develop gastroduodenal disorders. This implies near perfect adaptation to the niche and an ability to evade the human immune response. Of those infected, about 10% develop peptic ulceration, roughly 1% develop gastric adenocarcinoma and less than 0.1% MALT (mucosa-associated lymphoid tissue lymphoma). In 1994 the International Agency for Research on Cancer (IARC), a branch of the World Health Organization (WHO), classified it as a class I human carcinogen (Lee et al., 2008). *H. pylori* infection is the main risk factor in up to 92% of gastric cancers (González et al., 2012) and this cancer is the fourth most common and second most deadly cancer worldwide, with approximately 740,000 deaths per year. Studies have also associated *H. pylori* infection with diverse extragastric nonmalignant diseases (Banic et al., 2012).

In the absence of an effective vaccine, antibiotic treatment cures peptic ulcer disease and gastric MALT lymphoma permanently (when the treatment is given before the MALT lymphoma becomes autonomous) while gastric adenocarcinoma is difficult to prevent unless it is found at an early stage (Fukase et al., 2008). *H. pylori* infection can be difficult to treat and requires the combined intake of a proton pump inhibitor with amoxicillin and one of two antibiotics, clarithromycin or metronidazole.

Although *H. pylori* infection always causes a chronic active gastritis, the majority of infected individuals (~85%) remain asymptomatic throughout life. The factors influencing the evolution of *H. pylori* gastritis remain poorly understood and researchers continue to explore the complexities of infection, seeking to explain why some individuals have asymptomatic infection, whereas others experience clinical disease (Makola, 2007). Progression towards several divergent clinical outcomes depends on many variables, including bacterial genotype, host physiology and genetics, and environmental factors such as diet (Hunt, 1996, Makola, 2007).

The last two decades have seen major advances in unraveling the contribution of bacterial virulence factors, environmental exposures and host genetic factors in the pathogenesis of *H. pylori*-induced diseases. The specificity of *H. pylori* for the human host is the consequence of a series of adaptations that probably occurred many thousands of years ago reflected in regulatory, metabolic, and physiological features of the bacterium. The bacterium has developed a unique set of factors, actively supporting its successful survival and persistence in its natural hostile ecological niche, the human stomach, throughout the individual's life, unless treated. Its spiral shape and flagella allow it to corkscrew through the gastric mucus layer, and numerous adhesins enable selective adherence to the epithelium. One of the most efficient biological barriers against bacterial infection is the acidic pH (<2) of the gastric lumen. However, the mucus layer overlying gastric epithelial cells exhibits a pH gradient, ranging from about pH 2 at the luminal surface to between 5 and 6 at the epithelial surface (Talley et al., 1992). This human-specific bacillus is exquisitely adapted to survive within the hostile environment of the stomach. *H. pylori* possess multiple mechanisms for protection against gastric acid (Sachs, 2003); notably, 15% of its protein content comprises preformed cytoplasmic urease. To avoid the bactericidal activity of acid, *H. pylori* produce substantial amounts of cytosolic and cell surface-associated urease. When the external pH is less than 6.5, a specific channel opens in the bacterial cytoplasmic membrane, allowing ingress of urea (Weeks, 2000). The ammonia produced by urea hydrolysis neutralizes the periplasm, allowing maintenance of the cytoplasmic membrane potential (Weeks, 2000). In addition to facilitating survival and growth in acidic conditions, the ammonia produced via enzymatic degradation of urea is used for amino acid biosynthesis. The importance of ammonia in *H. pylori* metabolism and virulence is underlined by the presence of several alternative routes for ammonia production, via enzymatic degradation of diverse amides (aliphatic amidase, AmiE and formamidase, AmiF) as well as amino acids (Kusters, 2006).

To survive the host's immune defenses, *H. pylori* has evolved a multitude of unique characteristics and strategies. *H. pylori* shows extensive intrastrain and interstrain diversity, which assists the infecting agent, evade immune recognition. *H. pylori* is a microaerophilic bacterium that does not tolerate high oxygen conditions. In the human host, *H. pylori* is thought to be exposed to oxidative stress produced by the active immune response. To combat such forms of oxidative stress, *H. pylori* expresses several key components of bacterial oxidative stress resistance; these include the superoxide stress defense mediated via the iron-cofactored superoxide dismutase (SodB) and the peroxide stress

7

defense mediated via catalase (KatA) and alkyl hydroperoxide reductase (AhpC) (Kusters, 2006).

The majority of *H. pylori* strains express LPS that contains fucosylated oligosaccharide antigens that are structurally and immunologically closely related to human blood group antigens. These bacterial antigens mimic Lewis blood group antigens aiding molecular mimicry of host antigens and associated immune evasion (Correa, 2012). Additionally the innate immune recognition by several TLRs is attenuated for *H. pylori* (Backhed, F., et al. 2003; Lee, S.K., et al. 2003).

The adherence of *H. pylori* to the mucus layer of the gastric epithelium plays an important role in the initial colonization and persistence of the bacteria in the human stomach during decades or for an entire lifetime. *H. pylori* colonization of the stomach elicits humoral and cellular immune responses which in most cases do not result in bacterial clearance. Colonization of the gastric mucosa by *H. pylori* first results in the induction of an inflammatory response, predominantly of the Th1 type. The initial acute gastritis is followed by active chronic gastritis, which lasts for life if the infection is not treated. Nevertheless, *H. pylori*-positive subjects are mostly unaware of this inflammation due to the lack of clinical symptoms. It is estimated that *H. pylori*-positive patients have a 10 to 20% lifetime risk of developing ulcer disease and a 1 to 2% risk of developing distal gastric cancer (Kusters, 2006). The risk of development of these disorders in the presence of *H. pylori* infection depends on a variety of bacterial, host, and environmental factors that mostly relate to the pattern and severity of gastritis.

2. Infection prevalence

Infection with *H. pylori* is one of the most common bacterial infections in humans worldwide, with higher rates occurring in persons belonging to lower socioeconomic strata. Infection outcome is the result of a complex interplay between the host, bacterium and environmental factors. It is hypothesized thought that the loss of the natural balance between the two species may result in disease. In developing countries, the prevalence of *H. pylori* infection increases rapidly throughout the first two decades of life until upwards of 80 to 90% of the population is infected by early adulthood. Up to 15% to 20% of infected individuals will eventually develop severe gastrointestinal diseases. With such an extensive distribution, *H. pylori* infection represents a significant and important worldwide public health problem causing up to 7 million cases of *H. pylori*–induced diseases occurring annually (Parsonnett, 1998). Epidemiological studies indicate a decrease in infection rate (<50%) in much of the USA and western Europe and other pathologies like: gastroesophageal reflux disease, obesity and its associated diseases including type 2 diabetes and atopic and allergic diseases, including asthma have become more prevalent (Atherton and Balser, 2009; Carolina - Romo González, 2007). The rapidly declining prevalence of

H. pylori infection in industrialized world is thought to be caused by the reduced chances of childhood infection due to improved hygiene and sanitation and the active elimination of carriership via antimicrobial treatment. The incidence of new *H. pylori* infections among adults in the Western world is less than 0.5% per year (Kusters et al., 2006).

The mechanisms of *H. pylori* acquisition are poorly understood. Acquisition of *H. pylori* infection occurs predominantly in childhood, with more severe gastroduodenal diseases appearing mostly during adulthood. Gastro-oral, oral-oral and fecal-oral routes from human to human are the primary means of transmission. The likelihood of the transmission pathway in developing rural and developed urban areas appears to be different. In developed areas, person-to-person transmission within families appears to be dominant, while in the rural developing areas the transmission pathway appears to be more complex. Parents and siblings seem to play a major role in transmission. Reports have been shown that *H. pylori* isolates from children and their mothers often have the same genotype (Bauer and Meyer, 2011), supporting that infection primarily occurs during childhood via close contact to family members (e.g., via premastication of food by parents). Other possible transmission routes are: contaminated food or water, via domestic animals such as cats and sheep. The bacterium has been detected in saliva, supragingival and subgingival plaque, suggesting that these sites may be considered reservoirs for *H. pylori* not only in urease-positive patients, but in healthy volunteers and thus be involved in the reinfection of the stomach (Krasteva et al). Some studies show that dental plaque control and using new thoothbrush was associated with less gastric reinfection. Presently, no conclusive evidence of predominant transmission by any of these routes has been established.

3. Genus description and phylogeny

The genus *Helicobacter* belongs to the Epsilon subdivision of the Proteobacteria, order *Campylobacterales*, family *Helicobacteriaceae* (On, 2001). This family also includes the genera *Wolinella*, *Flexispira*, *Sulfurimonas*, *Thiomicrospira* and *Thiovulum*. There are currently over 20 formally validated *Helicobacter* species.The cultivation of *H. pylori* and the recognition of its clinical significance served to renew interest in bacteria associated with the gastrointestinal and hepato-biliary tracts of humans and other animals, many of which have now been identified as novel *Helicobacter* species. Helicobacters are non-spore-forming gram-negative bacteria, microaerophilic, and most cases are catalase and oxidase positive, and many species but not all are urease positive.

Colonization of the stomach or intestinal tract with Helicobacter species is ubiquitous in animal kingdom. These species can be subdivided into two major lineages, the gastric *Helicobacter* species and the enterohepatic (non-gastric) *Helicobacter* species, with high level of organ specificity.

The cellular morphology may be curved, spiral, or fusiform, typically 0.2 to 1.2 μm in diameter and 1.5 to 10.0 μm long. The spiral wavelength may vary with the age, the growth conditions, and the species identity of the cells. In old cultures or those exposed to air, cells may become coccoid. All helicobacters are motile by means of flagella. These basic characteristics of morphology and motility are thought to be advantageous to these organisms due to their localization in the mucous layer of the gastrointestinal tracts of humans and a variety of animals. Certain aspects of the ultrastructural detail of the helicobacters, e.g., sheathed flagella and surface urease, have been implicated in their ability to survive in hostile environments such as the acidic gastric mucosa and their ability to induce disease (Solnick and Vandamme, 2001).

H. pylori in vivo and under optimum in vitro conditions is an S-shaped bacterium with 1 to 3 turns, 0.5 ×5 μm in length, with a tuft of 5 to 7 polar sheathed flagella (Goodwin et al., 1985, Jones et al., 1985). This morphology has been correlated with maximum in vitro motility (Worku et al., 1999). The majority of helicobacters possess this basic morphology of an S shape with polar, sheathed flagella, though variations in size and the number of spirals/turns are seen. Generally it is considered that the spiral morphology and flagella are essential for colonization of gastric and intestinal mucus (Eaton et al., 1992).

H pylori possess unique features regarding colonization of the human gastric epithelium. It is localized in lower part of antrum (less acidic), but colonizes also corpus in low acidic conditions. The survival of *H. pylori* in the stomach is assured by production of high levels of urease. *H. pylori* is localized beneath the mucus layer, at the surface of epithelial cells where part of the population can be attached, but the great majority of bacteria are motile, using the mucus pH for chemotactic orientation (Schreiber et al., 2004). Recent data suggest that H. pylori can invade the gastric mucosal cells and repopulate the extracellular environment after complete elimination of the extracellular bacteria with antibiotics, suggesting it may be considered a facultative intracellular bacterium. This invasiveness may play a role in persistence and pathogenicity of the bacterium (reviewed in Dubois and Boren, 2007).

4. Pathogenicity-related factors of *H. pylori*

H. pylori exhibit both host tropism, exclusively colonizing humans and some primates, and tissue tropism, adhering only to the gastric epithelial lining of the antrum or staying in the gastric mucus layer. In the duodenum, gastric metaplasia is a pre-requisite for the presence of the bacterium, and reports exist of *H. pylori* colonization at distant sites of gastric metaplasia, such as in Meckel's diverticula containing gastric mucosa and in the rectum (Morris et al., 1989; Kestemberg et al., 1993).

In addition, *H. pylori* is not able to colonize areas of complete intestinal metaplasia in the gastric mucosa (Genta et al., 1996). The majority of the bacteria remain in the mucus layer, with a smaller proportion colonizing the gastric surface.

In the last three decades, remarkable progress has been made in the understanding of pathogenicity-related factors of *H. pylori* and their functional interaction with gastric epithelial cell components. These virulence-related factors are either secreted, membrane-associated, or translocated into the cytosol of host cells, where they can directly interfere with host cell functions. As a consequence of their different locations during the infection process, *H. pylori* is able to exploit a plurality of mechanisms to manipulate host cellular processes and to disregulate signaling cascades. The influence of *H. pylori* on these signaling pathways results in adherence, induction of proinflammatory responses through cytokine/chemokine release, apoptosis, proliferation, and a pronounced motogenic response as characterized *in vitro*. Taken together, these eventually result in persistent colonization, severe inflammation, disruption of the epithelial barrier function, and possibly gastric cancer. These effects originate from selective pathogen–host interactions. Many of these factors act cooperatively, eventually leading to a complex scenario of pathogenesis-related signaling events.

H. pylori has developed a unique set of factors, actively supporting its successful survival and persistence in its natural hostile ecological niche, the human stomach, throughout the individual's life, unless treated. In the human stomach, the vast majority of *H. pylori* cells are motile in the mucus layer lining, but a small percentage adheres to the epithelial cell surfaces. Adherence to the gastric epithelium is important for the ability of *H. pylori* to cause disease because this intimate attachment facilitates: (1) colonization and persistence, by preventing the bacteria from being eliminated from the stomach, by mucus turnover and gastric peristalsis; (2) evasion from the human immune system and (3) efficient delivery of proteins into the gastric cell, such as the CagA oncoprotein (Oleastro and Menard, 2013).

Cell-envelope components are the first points of contact between bacterial pathogens and the host. Many of the distinguishing properties of *H. pylori* are related to the constituents of this cellular compartment. Characterization of the cell envelope of *H. pylori* has identified a number of important features that distinguish it from other bacterial pathogens.

Like the cell envelopes of other gram-negative bacteria, that of *Helicobacter pylori* contains lipopolysaccharides (LPSs), which are a family of toxic phosphorylated glycolipids that are also termed endotoxins. It is an organic compound found in the outer leaflet of outer membranes which contributes to the structural integrity of the bacteria and protects the membrane and, as the main surface antigens (O-antigens) of gram-negative bacteria, plays an important role in the interaction of these bacteria with their environment and with higher organisms. Similar to other Gram-negative bacteria, the LPS of *H. pylori* is essential for the bacteria's survival. This family of compounds also harbors binding sites for antibodies and nonimmunoglubulin serum factors (Hols et al., 1996, Rietschel et al., 1990). Generally, LPSs possess a broad spectrum of endotoxic properties, e.g., pyrogenicity and lethal toxicity, which contribute to the pathogenic potential of gram-negative bacteria (Rietschel et al., 1991). Moreover, variation in the structure of the saccharide component of LPS may prevent efficient complement activation and phagocytosis, thereby contributing to the virulence of bacterial strains (Rietschel et al., 1990). Despite the established importance of LPSs in bacterial pathogenesis, those of *H. pylori* have received more limited attention compared with LPSs of other bacterial pathogens. Evidence has accumulated that, although possessing properties similar to those of other gram-negative bacteria, the LPSs of *H. pylori* also possess unique biological properties.

The LPS of *H. pylori* consists of an O-specific polysaccharide chain, a core oligosaccharide, and a lipid part called lipid A, embedded in the outer membrane. While LPS is often highly toxic for the host, that of *H. pylori* is low in activation of the host immunological responses (Muotiala et al., 1992). The most striking feature of the O antigen is the presence of extended chains with fucosylated and nonfucosylated *N*-acetyllactosamine units. The repeating units of the O side chains of LPS of *H. pylori* strains have been shown to mimic type 2 Lewis blood group antigens (Le^x and Le^y) in structure (Aspinall et al., 1996). Serological and structural studies have shown that *H. pylori* strains may also carry type 1 blood group determinants, namely, Le^a, H-1 (Le^d), and the type 1 chain precursor Le^c (Monteiro et al., 1998). Many α-2-fucosyltransferases are involved in the addition of fucose to create the A, B, H, and Lewis blood group antigens. These include the products of the H, Se, A, B, X, and Le genes. In the case of Le^a and Le^b antigens, Le^a is created by fucosylation of the type 1 precursor by the product of the Le gene whereas Le^b is created by the fucosylation of the type 1 precursor to form the H type 1 antigen followed by fucosylation by the product of the Le gene to give the Le^b antigen. A similar pathway is used in the biosynthesis of the Le^x and Le^y blood group antigens, except both are formed from the type 2 precursor. The type 2 precursor is fucosylated by either the product of the Le or X genes forming Le^x or the precursor is fucosylated by either the Se or H gene product to form the H type 2 antigen and then fucosylated further by either the Le or X gene product to form Le^y. Thus, the pathway is made up of various enzymes competing for the same substrate. *H. pylori* may use similar enzymes to synthesize Lewis antigens (Solnick and Vandamme, 2001).

Lewis-like antigens are also expressed on gastric epithelial cells (Monteiro et al., 2000) It was hypothesized that these *H. pylori* LPS Lewis-like antigens could play a role in adherence to gastric epithelial

17

cells in a Lewis-antigen-dependent manner, more specifically via Lex. Moreover, since they undergo phase variation and antigenic variation within a single strain, this would provide the bacteria with a dynamic adherent phenotype (Edwards et al., 2000; Monteiro et al., 1998; Appelmelk et al., 1998). Several studies support the role of LPS as an adherence factor of *H. pylori*. In one study, a monoclonal antibody that inhibited *H. pylori* adherence to gastric epithelial cells by up to 75% was shown to target the LPS possibly through the O-antigen Lex portion (Osaki et al., 1998). More recently, the receptor recognized by the O-antigen side-chain of *H. pylori* LPS was identified as being a host β-galactoside-binding lectin, galectin-3 (Fowler et al., 2006). The study also showed that expression of galectin-3 is up regulated by gastric epithelial cells following adherence of *H. pylori*, suggesting that, in addition to colonization, this lectin also plays a role in the host response to infection. However other reports suggests that Lewis-like antigens seem to only have a limited role in bacterial adherence, which is most likely overcome by the strong adherence phenotype mediated by *H. pylori* adhesins (Odenbreit et al., 2002; Mahdavi et al., 2003).

Little information is available on the effects of *H. pylori* LPS on epithelial cells, indicating a yet undefined role in the *H. pylori*-infected epithelium as well. However, it has been suggested that *H. pylori* LPS might be a TLR2 agonist in gastric MKN45 cells, contributing to the

18

activation of nuclear factor kappa B (NF-κB) and chemokine expression independently of the canonical LPS receptor TLR4 (Smith et al., 2003).

Gram-negative bacterial outer membranes mediate the interaction with the surrounding environment. For *H. pylori* to survive and persist in the gastric mucosa, adaptation of the outer membrane could be expected. Comparative analysis of two complete *H. pylori* genome sequences has confirmed the presence of large families of integral outer membrane proteins that represent approximately 4% of each strain's coding potential. The use of outer membrane proteins as adhesins may represent an adaptation to the gastric environment, where the acidic conditions would likely depolymerize any polymeric pilus structure. A similar adaptation may be the encasement of the flagellum of *H. pylori* by a sheath with a composition similar to that of the outer membrane, an organization that may also protect the polymeric flagellar structure (Alm et al., 2000).

Analysis of the three completed *H pylori* genomes (strains 26695, J99, and HPAG1) has confirmed the presence of five major outer membrane protein (OMPs) families. The largest family is Family 1, comprised of the Hop (for *H. pylori* OMP, 21 members) and Hor (for Hop related, 12 members) proteins. Families 2 and 3 comprise the Hof (for *Helicobacter* OMP, 8 members) and Hom (for *Helicobacter* outer membrane, 4 members) proteins, respectively. Families 4 and 5 are composed of iron-regulated OMPs (6 members) and efflux pump OMPs (3 members), respectively.

Other OMPs (~10 members) were not included in these families (Alm et al., 2000).

Members of the large Hop (*Helicobacter* outer membrane protein) family were the first characterized OMPs in *H pylori*. Several OMPs in the Hop family have been reported to act as adhesion molecules including the blood group antigen binding adhesin (BabA), which was the first identified adhesin in *H. pylori* and is the best-characterized adhesin-receptor interaction in *H pylori*, sialic acid binding adhesin (SabA), adherence-associated lipoprotein (AlpA and AlpB), outer membrane inflammatory protein (OipA), and HopZ.

Lewis b antigen (Le^b) and related fucosylated ABO blood group antigens are recognized by BabA, whereas sialyl-Lewis x and sialyl-Lewis a antigens (sLe^x and sLe^a) are recognized by SabA. BabA-mediated adhesion of *H. pylori* to gastric epithelial cells might enhance CagA translocation and the induction of inflammation (Ishijima et al., 2011). Furthermore, triple-positive clinical *H. pylori* isolates (BabA$^+$, VacAs1$^+$, CagA$^+$) show greater colonization densities, elevated levels of gastric inflammation and a higher incidence of intestinal metaplasia in *H. pylori*-infected patients as compared to VacAs1$^+$, CagA$^+$ double-positive variants (Rad et al., 2002). Epidemiologically, triple-positive strains are correlated with the highest incidence of ulceration and gastric cancer (Gerhard et al., 1999).

Members of the Hop family share highly similar or identical sequences at their amino and carboxyl termini and include porins and several known or predicted *H. pylori* adhesins which promote binding to the gastric epithelium. In addition, another OMP from the third family, HomB, was shown to be involved in *H. pylori* adherence and associated with with IL-8 secretion *in vitro* (Oleastro et al., 2008). The level of the expression of *H. pylori* OMPs can be altered and regulated by several mechanisms, of which the most important are: gene conversion and gene duplication, regulation by phase variation and allelic variation (Oleastro and Menard, 2013).

Although bacterial adherence is crucially important for *H. pylori* pathogenesis, data showing direct effects of the above adherence factors on signaling pathways are scarce. This indicates that canonical adhesins may not directly activate signaling, but rather mediate a tight interaction between *H. pylori* and the host target cell, probably paving the way for additional bacterial factors to interact with their cognate receptors (Posselt et al., 2013).

In addition to OMPs and adhesins, flagellin and LPS have been widely investigated to address their role in *H. pylori* pathogenesis. In general, flagellin and LPS are important factors in many other bacterial infections, but it is unclear to what extent both factors contribute to *H.*

pylori-induced signaling events. In contrast to the flagellin of other bacterial pathogens, *H. pylori* flagellin has only a very low capacity to stimulate toll-like receptor 5 (TLR5)-dependent interleukin-8 (IL-8) release (Lee et al., 2003). This has been confirmed by the finding that purified *H. pylori* flagellin is a poor ligand for TLR5 (Andersen-Nissen et al., 2005).

There is considerable interest in identifying *virulence factors* that are *Helicobacter pylori* disease specific (eg, related to duodenal ulcer and not gastric cancer). Several virulence factors such as the *cag* pathogenicity island, *vacA*, *oipA* and *babA* have been described and have been associated with an increase in the risk of both gastric cancer and duodenal ulcer disease (Zang et al., 2008). They have also been associated with an increase in mucosal inflammation which is thought to underlie both duodenal ulcers and gastric cancer. However, reports on the clinical predictive value of putative virulence factor status and disease outcomes are controversial, at least in all ethnic groups (Chiarini et al. 2008; Dossumbekova et al., 2006; Douraghi et al., 2008; Erzin et al., 2006; Gomes et al. 2008; Hocker & Hohenberger, 2003; Lu et al. 2005). Different putative virulence factors might undergo a continuously evolving mechanism as an approach to bacterial adaptation to the changing host environment during infection (Marshall et al., 1998; Alvi et al., 2007).

Putative virulence genes are generally classified into three categories: (i) strain-specific genes such as *cag pathogenicity island* (*cag* PAI) genes and genes located in the plasticity region (e.g. *jhp0947* and *dupA* genes); (ii) phase-variable genes (e.g. *oipA, sabA, sabB, babB, babC*) and (iii) genes with variable structures/ genotypes (e.g. vacA) (Yamaoka, 2008).

Cag pathogenicity island (*cag* PAI), a 40-kb DNA segment integrated in the *H. pylori* chromosome may be present, absent, or disrupted and thus nonfunctional. It is most commonly present and functional, being associated with enhanced virulence as measured by mucosal inflammation (Censini, S., et al. 1996). The cag PAI DNA segment contains genes constituting a type IV secretion apparatus (T4SS), as well as the *cagA* gene that encodes highly immunogenic CagA protein, with a molecular weight between 120 and 140 kDa (Higashi, 2002, Atherton and Blaser, 2009). The *cag*-T4SS represents a needle-like structure (also called T4SS pilus) protruding from the bacterial surface and connecting the cytoplasm of bacterial and host epithelial cells. An antigenically variable, acid-stable structural protein *H. pylori* (CagY) coats the "syringe," conferring stability and allowing evasion from the host immune response. The *cag*-T4SS apparently does not inject its effector protein CagA randomly into target cells, but uses the α5β1 integrin as a cellular receptor for the pilus-associated adhesin CagL (Kwok, T., et al. 2007). CagL is the only *cag*-PAI encoded protein carrying an RGD sequence, which is present in certain extracellular matrix proteins and known as a typical integrin/ligand interaction motif (Takagi, 2004). Upon translocation, CagA is immediately tyrosine-phosphorylated at a variable number of so-called EPIYA (Glu-Pro-Ile-Tyr-Ala) motifs by kinases of the Src and c-Abl family (Backert, 2001; Poppe, 2007; Shiota, 2010), leading to different effects on cellular signaling and differing risks of disease (Higashi, H., et al. 2002, Argent, R.H., et al. 2004; 2008; Yamaoka, Y., et al. 1999; Basso, D., et al. 2008). These EPIYA motifs can be repeated within the protein's variable region (Argent et al., 2005), and are defined as EPIYA-A, -B, -C, and -D according to the amino acids surrounding them. Species of nearby CagA proteins almost always contain EPIYA-A and EPIYA-B sites, followed by one to three repetitions of EPIYA-C in the *H. pylori* Western-type isolates (ABC, ABCC, and ABCCC) or one EPIYA-D site in East Asian-type isolates (ABD).

The east-Asian-type CagA, containing EPIYA-D segments, exhibits a stronger binding affinity for Src homology-2 domain-containing phosphatase (SHP)2 and a greater ability to induce morphological changes in epithelial cells than Western-type CagA, which contains segments EPIYA-C segments (Higashi, H., et al. 2002, Argent, et al.. 2008; Delahay, R.M., et al. 2008, Shiota, 2010). Another recent study showed that *H. pylori* strains possessing east-Asian-type CagA induce higher amounts of interleukin-8 (IL-8) from gastric

24

epithelial cells than those possessing Western-type CagA. Accordingly, east-Asian strains are believed to be more virulent than Western strains, and this might be the reason why the incidences of gastric cancer are relatively higher in east-Asian countries than in Europe, North America and Australia (Atherton and Blaser, 2009; Shiota, 2010). Hence, determination of the number of EPIYA motifs within the *cagA* variable region in clinical *H. pylori* isolates is more important than the mere detection of the *cagA* and can be useful in predicting the bacteria's pathogenic activity.

Besides CagA translocation, the T4SS is also involved in the production of chemokines, such as IL-8, process mediated by the combinatorial activation of the host cell transcription factors NF-κB and AP-1.Phosphorylation and subsequent activation of these factors is dependent on the intracellular pattern recognition factor NOD-1 (nucleotide-binding oligomerization domain-containing protein 1), which is known to recognize universal bacterial components such as peptidoglycan. Indeed, peptidoglycan was suggested to be translocated into the host cell in a T4SS-dependent manner, thereby, inducing the activation of NF-κB via NOD-1 (Bauer and Meyer, 2011).

CagA interacts with a large set of host proteins in phosphorylation-dependent and independent ways and is considered a bacterial oncoprotein that exerts multiple effects on host signal transduction pathways, the cytoskeleton and cellular junctions (Hatakeyama, 2004).

CagA appears to be centrally important in *H. pylori*–induced gastric carcinogenesis, regardless of inflammation status (Atherton and Balser, 2009).

Adhesion molecules act in conjunction with factors from the *cag* PAI in order to highjack several host cell processes including altered transcription, cytoskeletal rearrangements, opening of cell-to-cell junctions, onset of inflammation and others (Backert et al., 2011).

Duodenal ulcer–promoting gene A (*dupA*) is so named because originally it was reported to be rare (9%) among patients with gastric cancer and common (42%) among patients with duodenal ulcer (Zhang et al., 2008). Several studies have shown associations with both conditions, as might be expected for a factor associated with increased IL-8 release and gastritis in vivo (Gomes et al., 2008; Argent et al., 2007; Zhang et al. 2008). The *dupA* gene is thought to be a homolog of the *virB4* gene and is located in plasticity region of the *H. pylori* genome It may be the ATPase of an as yet uncharacterized T4SS (Lu et al., 2005).

Adhesion is a prerequisite for both *H. pylori* colonization and disease induction, and some strains adhere better than others to epithelial cells (Gerhard et al. 1999). Intensive research in recent years has demonstrated that *H. pylori* encode a broad set of various adhesion factors. The complete genome sequence revealed a family of more than 30 outer membrane proteins (OMPs) in *H. pylori*, that have been divided

26

into Hop (*Helicobacter* outer membrane porins) and Hor (hop-related) subgroups. The Hop family of proteins includes several well described adhesins of *H. pylori* such as BabA, SabA, AlpA/B, HopZ and OipA. The repertoire of functional adhesins includes appears to have been driven by human evolution (Atherton and Blaser, 2009).

The cellular adhesin most closely and consistently associated with disease is blood group antigen–binding adhesin A (BabA; encoded by *babA2*). This recognizes Lewis Blood Group epitopes on epithelial cells and is often found in *H. pylori* strains associated with gastric cancer (Gerhard, M., et al. 1999).

OipA (outer inflammatory protein A), encoded by the *hopH* gene, was initially identified as a surface protein that promoted IL-8 production in a T4SS-independent fashion (Yamaoka et al., 2000). *hopH* gene is an inflammation-related gene located approximately 100 kb from the cag PAI on the *H. pylori* chromosome (Ayala et al., 2008). *H. pylori* could be divided into two types (functional and nonfunctional) in relation to the *oipA gene*, based on their ability to induce production of the proinflammatory cytokine, IL-8. The *oip*A gene is regulated by slipped-strand repair mechanism based on the number of CT dinucleotide repeats in the 5 region of the gene. These types of repair mechanisms have evolved in bacterial pathogens to increase the frequency of phenotypic variation in genes involved in critical interactions with their hosts (Yamaoka et al., 2000). The presence of *oipA* has been shown to clearly enhance production of IL-8 *in vitro* but only in the presence of the *cag*PAI (Odenbreit et al., 2009). OipA expression by *H. pylori* was shown to be significantly associated with the presence of duodenal ulcers and gastric cancer, high *H. pylori* density, and severe neutrophil infiltration (Yamaoka et al., 2006).

OipA possibly interferes directly with signal transduction pathways that are predominantly activated by T4SS/CagA factors. This might indicate that OipA contributes to T4SS-dependent cellular responses, either through the direct activation of a yet unidentified receptor or indirectly through mediating tight adhesion between *H. pylori* and the host cell, leading to stronger T4SS/CagA-mediated signaling.

The vacuolating toxin, VacA is a paradigmatic type-V-secreted bacterial toxin that contributes to the establishment of successful infection and virulence in multiple ways. Similar to CagA, it has been shown to be responsible for epithelial ulceration (Bauer and Meyer, 2011). Virtually all strains of *H. pylori* possess the gene *vacA*, and nearly all produce a VacA protein (Cover, 1994). However, only about 40% make the most active form. Two regions of marked sequence diversity are distinguishable within the *vacA* gene. The *s* region (encodes the signal peptide) is present as *s1* or *s2* allele, while the *m* region (mid region) can be *m1* or *m2*. The combination of the allele mosaic from the *s* and *m* region determines the production of vacuolating cytotoxin and is associated to the bacteria's pathogenicity. The strains harbored *vacA* *s1m1* have been strongly associated to increased virulence and greater epithelial gastric damage and ulceration than *s2m2* strains (Sicinschi et al., 2008, Vega et al., 2010). Thus, *cagA*-positive and *vacA s1m1* genotypes are associated to high risk of gastric cancer (Panayotopoulou et al., 2007).

VacA is a protein toxin, formed by monomers of ~90 kDa, able to induce cytoplasmic vacuoles in eukaryotic cells in culture. Cytoplasmic vacuoles are also present in vivo in the gastric epithelium of *H. pylori* colonized patients. After cell internalization, VacA localizes in the endocytic-endosomal compartment from which vacuoles originate. It has been reported that VacA may act as a channel-forming toxin and it has also been proposed that VacA channels play a direct role in cell vacuolation.

Besides its ability to induce the vacuolation of epithelial cells in vitro, VacA can also promote apoptosis of gastric epithelial cells by targeting mitochondria (Chiozzi et al., 2009); this in turn enhances the hyper proliferative response, altering the balance of gastric homeostasis, which changes gastric epithelial cell turnover and permits the persistence of mutated cells. Studies suggest that these processes may promote carcinogenesis (Galmiche et al., 2000). Moreover, the immunosuppressive properties of VacA may play an important role in enabling *H. pylori* to persistently colonize the human host (Bauer and Meyer, 2011).

One problem that has possibly complicated identification of definite disease-specific *H. pylori* virulence factors is the considerable geographic diversity in the prevalence of *H. pylori* virulence factors. For example, in some regions, (ie, East Asia) the vast majority of strains have similar if not identical patterns of virulence factors such that potentially important factors can best be identified in regions where there is considerable diversity among strains. For example, the associations between the *cag* pathogenicity island, *vacA*, *oipA* and *babA* and enhanced mucosal inflammation, gastric cancer and peptic ulcer were identified and confirmed in Western countries where there is considerable strain diversity (Zhang, 2008). How these factors result in disease is becoming better understood, although the benefit to *H. pylori* of possessing them remains less clear. One possibility is that the epithelial changes *H. pylori* causes (directly and perhaps also through inflammation) allow increased nutrient delivery to the bacterium. Alternatively, or additionally, these host interactions may induce niche modification, resulting in better conditions for survival of *H. pylori* or worse conditions for survival of competing bacteria (Atherton and Blaser, 2009).

H. pylori exhibits extraordinary allelic diversity and genetic variability (Sicinschi et al., 2008), generated through an elevated rate of point mutations, intragenomic and intergenomic recombination (Suerbaum and Josenhans, 2007), phenomena facilitated by the presence of reactive oxygen species (ROS) and reactive nitrogen species (RNS) produced from inflammatory lesions induced by the *H. pylori* infection. This complex environment propitiates a second-order selection that implies variation in mutator genes, creating a non-linear diversification system (Atherton and Blaser, 2009). The fact that virulence factors in *H. pylori* are linked to disease implies that they are a fixed characteristic, but this is not the case and genotype variations can occur through genetic rearrangements (Atherton and Blaser, 2009) that eliminates particular immune-stimulating genetic regions (*cag* PAI) or causes variations in potential immune-stimulating molecules (number of EPIYA repetitions in CagA (Suerbaum and Josenhans, 2007), probably reflecting the local selection of *H. pylori* particular phenotypes (Atherton and Blaser, 2009) as an escape recourse to the immune response of the host induced by environmental pressures.

Within the gastric niche, genetic and phenotypic diversity within the resident *H. pylori* population may exist, reflecting the dynamics of the host-microbial cross talk. Genetic changes within the genome of the colonizing strain, accumulated during the years of infection, may give rise to different clones. Additionally, subpopulations of *H. pylori* can arise from two or more unrelated sources due to multiple infections of the host. The presence of subclones with various genotypes that allow bacteria to be more or less pathogenic maximizes the opportunities for survival, persistence, and spread. At any given time, there is an expansion of the subtype that best adapts to the host. Given the facts that *H. pylori* infection is chronic and that the organism maintains its niche in a continuously changing habitat, this capacity could be of major importance. Disease occurs when this subtle balance is disturbed, for instance, due to changes in the environment or in host mucosal barrier functions that render the host more susceptible to virulent subtypes (Nilsson et al., 2003).

5. Correlation between *cag* PAI status and clinical outcome

Helicobacter pylori infection is associated with a variety of outcomes ranging from seemingly asymptomatic coexistence to peptic ulcer disease and gastric cancer. The *cag* pathogenicity island (PAI) contains genes associated with a more aggressive phenotype and has been suggested to be a determinant of severe disease outcome. Reports suggest that *H. pylori* strains have to carry intact *cag* PAIs in order to be associated with the development of severe disease. Strains that have internal deletions in the *cag* PAI have reduced virulence and could be compared to *cag* PAI-negative strains (Nilsson et al., 2003).

The *cagA* gene has served as a marker for the *cag* PAI, present in over 50% of the *H. pylori* strains, encodes for the CagA protein one of the main determinants of pathogenicity associated to infection by *H. pylori*. Studies suggest that infection with *cagA* positive *H. pylori* strains induces a marked inflammatory response, with a great density of polymorphonuclear cells in the gastric mucosa and high levels of serum tumor necrosis alpha-factor and gastrin, which are seen as markers of inflammation in *H.pylori* infection, when compared with the *cagA* negative strains (Gatti et al., 2006). However, studies have provided more inconsistent results. Miehlke et al. demonstrated that up to 80% of subjects without ulcer disease in Texas (USA) were infected with *H. pylori* strains that possessed *cag*A gene. In China and Japan, cagA-positive strains are nearly universally present and not associated with disease complications. In children, infection with *cagA*-positive strains has not been consistently associated with peptic ulcer disease. These findings suggest that polymorphism of the *cag* A gene can be relevant, but the presence of other possible *H. pylori* virulence genes may also be (Lima et al., 2010).

Another of the *cag*-PAI genes is *cag* E, located in the right half of the cag-PAI. Sozzi et al. (2005) and Ikenoue et al. (2001) have suggested that this gene is a more accurate marker of an intact cag- PAI than other *cag* genes.

In Europe, *cagA*-positive *H pylori* has been reported to account for 60% to 70% of *H pylori* strains (Peters et al., 2001), while reports from East Asian countries have shown that more than 90% of *H pylori* strains are *cagA* positive irrespective of the disease presentation (Saribasak et al., 2004).

CagA-positive isolates do not necessarily have to be *cag* PAI positive, and vice versa. Censini et al. first identified strains with partially deleted *cag* PAIs. The molecular mechanism of these genetic rearrangements was explained by incorporation of an insertion element, IS*605*, in the *cag* PAI (Censini, 1996). Some *H. pylori* strains contain only parts of the *cag* PAI and not the whole set of 27 genes. Strains with partially deleted *cag* PAIs may be *cagA* positive or negative, and even though they represent an intermediate form (Salama et al., 2000).

6. Correlation between circulating CagA antibodies and cag status

Infection with *H pylori* elicits a systemic, strong and polymorphic humoral immune response. CagA is the important pathologic marker with a high immunogenic response (Herbrink & van Doorn 2000).

Several studies have shown that the detection of CagA antibodies in serum samples does not always correlate with the presence or absence of the *cagA* gene in the corresponding *H. pylori* isolate (Cover et al., 1995; Enroth et al., 1999). This observation can be explained by three alternative mechanisms. First, a mixed population of both *cagA*-positive and *cagA*-negative strains is present in the gastric environment, although only *cagA*-negative clones have been isolated and analyzed. Second, the patient could have been colonized by a *cagA*-positive strain at an earlier stage of the infection. The isolated strain has subsequently lost the *cag*

PAI, or *cag*-negative isolates in a mixed infection could have clonally expanded and obliterated the *cag*-positive strains. Third, the strain carries and expresses the *cagA* gene but other genes in the *cag* PAI are deleted or nonfunctional. If the components of the type IV secretion machinery are absent, no secretion of the CagA antigen will occur and antibodies may not be produced (Nilssen et al., 2003).

7. Correlation between circulating CagA antibodies and clinical outcome

Serological tests are non-invasive methods that have value for the diagnosis of *H. pylori* infection because they are both simple and convenient. Although the serum antibody response to *H. pylori* depends on both the characteristics of the strain and the host response, it can provide clues in predicting the severity of *H. pylori*-associated diseases.

Previous studies have reported the anti-CagA antigen is highly associated with gastric cancer and peptic ulcer (Rocha et al., 2000; Parsonnet et al., 1997), thus the ***CagA titre*** is considered an important marker clinically. Yang et al (2001) reported significantly higher serum anti-CagA IgG-positive rates in patients with duodenal ulcer (90.8%), gastric cancer (89.7%), gastric ulcer (83.2%) and chronic atrophic gastritis (70.5%) than in patients with chronic superficial gastritis (55.4%), and CagA positive rates in patients with intestinal metaplasia, atypical hyperplasia and gastric cancer were significantly higher than in patients with chronic gastritis. In contrast, infection with CagA-positive *H. pylori* is frequently found not only in duodenal ulcers but in chronic atrophic gastritis in the Japanese population.

Deguchi et al. (2004) reported serum anti-CagA IgG-positive in only 48.3% (14/29) of the cancers patients, the reason may be due in part to the CagA EIA kit used. As the EIA kit originated from Italy, the sensitivity for CagA detection may be dependent on the strain diversity between Asian and Western countries.

The anti-*H. pylori* CagA-Ig G antibodies are assessed for determining if a person was infected/is infected with a *cag*A positive isolate. These antibodies can persist four years after infection and have the advantage of detecting retrospective infection (Chien et al., 2005) this fact being particularly useful in gastric cancer patients for correlating the association of the malignant disease with *H.pylori* (Chan et al, 2009). The disadvantage of this marker is that the presence of the respective antibodies cannot differentiate present from past infections and it cannot be used for checking the eradication of *H. pylori* infection, the rapid urease test performed from gastric mucosa, urea breath test or less invasively fecal antigen test being more reliable to achieve this task. Ilie et al. (2011) study regarding the possible correlations between the presence of *H. pylori* CagA-IgG antibodies and the severity of clinical and endoscopical findings showed that from the cases resistant to first line therapy, 21 patients with gastritis proved to be positive for anti *H.*

pylori CagA-IgG antibodies and 4 negative. The patients exhibited significantly higher serum anti-CagA IgG-positive (>100 arbU/ml) (Ilie et al., 2011). In the same study, a number of 35 cases of bleeding ulcers were anti-CagA positive, 15 (42%) of them being also NSAID (Nonsteroidal anti-inflammatory drugs) positive. Seven cases of bleeding ulcers were cag A negative, 4 from them being NSAID positive. The cag A positive, NSAID negative exhibited high titres (>60 arbU/ml) in comparison with cag A positive, NSAID positive that had low titres (Fig. 1).

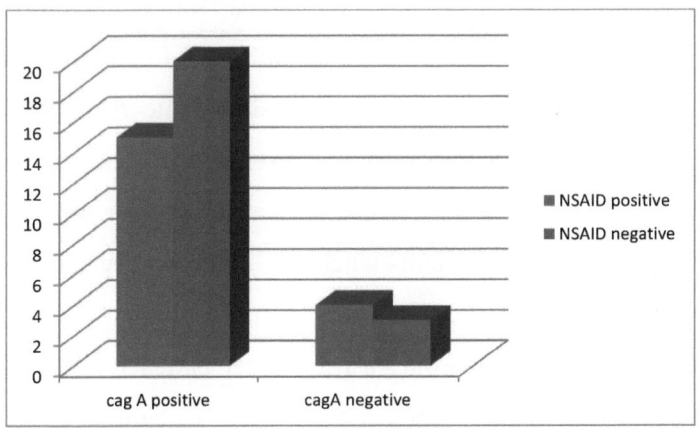

Figure 1. Distribution of bleeding gastroduodenal ulcers in function of anti-CagA positivity and NSAID administration

Anti-CagA IgG antibodies can persist up to four years, being present also in patients with non cardia gastric cancer and past infection of *H. pylori*, proving the implication of *H. pylori* in the pathogenesis of noncardia gastric cancer. Also, another drawback is that in many cases biopsy for *H.pylori* in gastric cancer patients is negative (rapid urease test or histology) because of glandular atrophy and intestinal metaplasia, which are considered precursors of gastric cancer. These are environments in which *H. pylori* might disappear. Moreover, the distribution of atrophy and intestinal metaplasia is uneven, and that might also affect the sensitivity of the various biopsy sites. In these cases anti-cagA IgG antibiodies presence proves the infection with *H. pylori*. The most appropriate biopsy site for *H. pylori* detection in gastric cancer patients, according to the previous studies, is from upper body greater curvature, where atrophy or intestinal metaplasia is relatively uncommon (1%-2%). Atrophy and intestinal metaplasia initiate from the antrum, due to chronic *H. pylori* infection, and extend to the corpus along the lesser curvature (Chan et al., 2009). This is in contrast with non-ulcer dyspepsia or peptic ulcer patients where the antral biopsy specimens had excellent sensitivity and specificity for H. pylori (over 90%). Ilie et al. reported that 83,33% noncardia gastric cancer patients were anti-CagA positive. (Fig. 2). All cases comprised the four categories of Borrmann classification (Fig. 3-4).

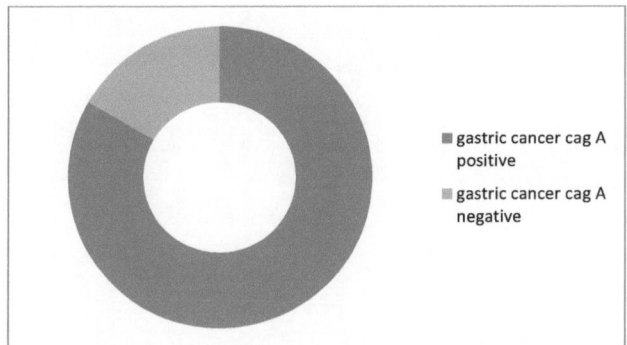

Figure 2. Predominance of anti- cagA Ig G positive in gastric cancer cases

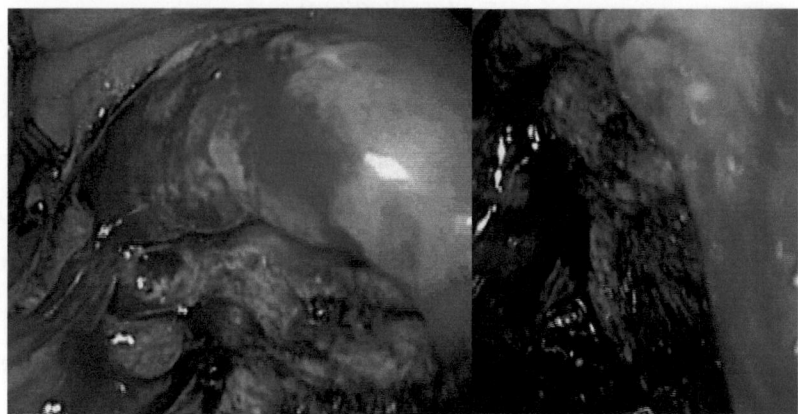

Fig. 3. Images of vegetant-ulcerative with spontaneous bleeding tumor (type II in Borrmann classification)

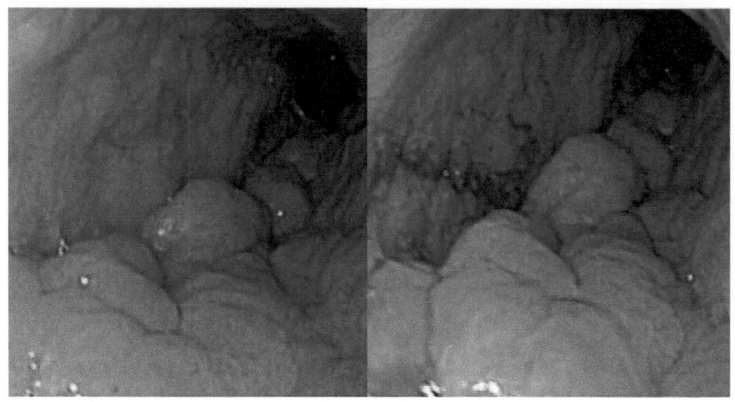

Figure 4. Images of diffuse infiltrative tumor (type IV in Borrmann classification)

Previous studies have shown that the anti-*H. pylori* Ig G antibodies synthetized routinely may persist maximum two years, thus detection of anti-CagA antibodies may represent a simple and rapid method for diagnosis of previous long-term *H. pylori* infections. Study of Ilie et al. indicated that out of the total number of patients positive for anti-*H. pylori* CagA-IgG antibodies, 17 were positive for the rapid urease test (RUT), showing active infection and 8 negative, proving a past infection. Thus the presence of anti-Cag A-IgG antibodies is an important marker for retrospective infection with *H. pylori* in non cardial gastric cancer. The patients with positive anti-CagA IgG and *H. pylori* infection (RUT positive) exhibited high levels of antibodies in comparison with past infection of *H. pylori* with low titres (5-40 arbU/ml). Also, from the 7 cases of gastric polyps, 5 were positive for anti-cag A IgG, the highest titres being registered in case of patients with multiple polyps. The p-value calculated by T-Test regarding the association between the anti-CagA IgG antibodies and different clinical or bacteriological parameters, i.e.: resistant cases to first line therapy for *H. pylori*, bleeding gastro-duodenal ulcers, non cardia gastric cancer and gastric polyps was 0.02, which is statistically significant (Fig. 5).

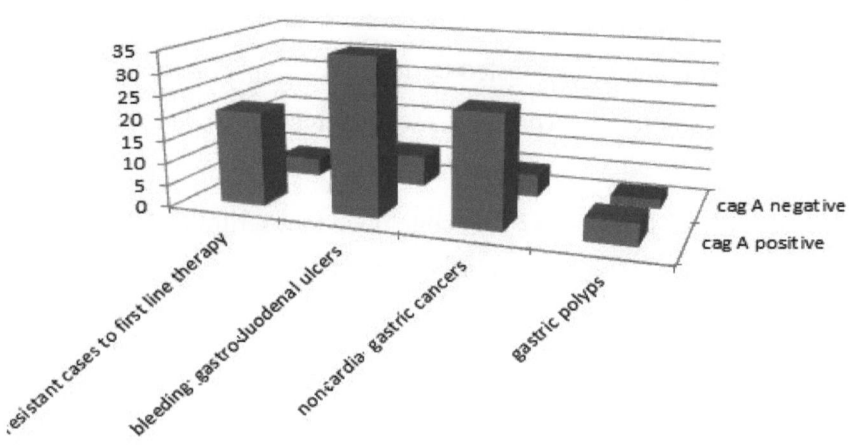

Fig. 5. Relation between selected cases (resistance cases to first line therapy for H. pylori, bleeding gastroduodenal ulcers, noncardia gastric cancer and gastric polyps) and cag A Ig G antibodies

The study of Ilie et al. (2011) suggest that detection of anti-CagA IgG antibodies in patients with positive biopsy for *H. pylori* indicates the need for treating *H. pylori* infection and eradication survey, one month after treatment (by fecal antigen or urea breath test). Several reports are indicating the potential of preventing gastric cancer by *H. pylori* eradication-screening and treating all positive patients (Malfertheiner et al., 2005). The results of these studies remain to be established, but the presence of anti-CagA antibiodies strengthens the necessity of treatment of *H. pylori* infection (non-invasively tested by fecal antigen test or urea breath test). For the antibiotic resistant cases, with *H. pylori* detected one month after treatment (when tested by urea breath test or fecal antigen), culture and antibiotic susceptibility assay is recommended (Ilie et al., 2011).

The study of Ilie et al. (2011) concluded that serum anti-CagA IgG titre is an important marker with clinically value. The researchers reported that the serum CagA is significantly associated with resistance to the first line of antibiotics for *H. pylori*, bleeding gastroduodenal ulcers, noncardia gastric cancer and gastric polyps. Higher serum anti-CagA IgG-positive levels were registered in *H.pylori* infections with antibiotic resistance to first line therapy, bleeding gastroduodenal ulcers, NSAID negative and noncardia gastric cancer. Additionaly a high percentage (42%) of the Cag A positive, bleeding cases were also NSAID positive, pointing out that in gastroduodenal bleeding ulcers associated with NSAID, *H. pylori* should be also tested, the summing of these two factors increasing the risk of hemorrhage.

8. Clinical manifestations of Helicobacter pylori infection

H. pylori infection is associated with divergent clinical outcomes that range from simple asymptomatic gastritis to serious conditions such as peptic ulcer disease and gastric neoplasia. The key determinants of these outcomes are the severity and distribution of the *H. pylori*-induced gastritis. Patients with antral predominant gastritis, the most common form of *H. pylori* gastritis, are predisposed to duodenal ulcers, whereas patients with corpus-predominant gastritis and multifocal atrophy are more likely to have gastric ulcers, gastric atrophy, intestinal metaplasia and, ultimately, gastric carcinoma (Suerbaum and Michetti, 2002).

Acute Gastritis. *H. pylori* is usually acquired in childhood although new infection of adults can occur. Initial colonization by *H. pylori* leads to acute gastritis . Acute infection may be associated with a transient mild illness characterized by epigastric pain, vomiting and indigestion but may pass unnoticed. Most symptoms usually resolve within 2 weeks. *H. pylori* infection causes a neutrophilic gastritis and then a gradual infiltration by all classes of inflammatory cells, predominantly lymphocytes occurs. Gastric acid secretion is often reduced and this transient hypochlorhydria may be caused by a direct toxic effect of *H. pylori* or by inflammatory cytokines such as interleukin 1, which inhibits acid secretion. Approximately 4 weeks after the initial infection, antibodies against *H. pylori* appear in the blood. Clinically, an acute *H. pylori* infection can be diagnosed by the presence of a positive urea breath test and negative IgG anti-*H. pylori* antibodies.

Chronic Gastritis Chronic *H. pylori* gastritis affects two-thirds of the world's population and is one of the most common chronic inflammatory disorders of humans. The major clinical associations with chronic *H. pylori* gastritis are peptic ulcer disease and, less commonly, gastric cancer and MALT lymphoma. Chronic gastritis is an inflammatory condition of the gastric mucosa that may affect different regions of the stomach and exhibit varying degrees of mucosal damage. The presence of *H. pylori* in the stomach is always associated with tissue damage and histologic findings of active and chronic gastritis. Typically, although present in both the corpus and antrum, the organisms are usually more common in the antrum(antrum and body – 80%, antrum only – 8%, body only – 10%). Histologically, an inflammatory infiltrate of lymphocytes and plasma cells is present within the lamina propria. Active inflammation is signified by the presence of neutrophils within the glandular and surface epithelial layer. Varying degrees of active inflammation can be detected. Lymphoid aggregates are frequently observed within the mucosa. Lymphoid follicles represent an immune response to the organism, and are composed of aggregates of

44

lymphocytes and other lymphoid cells associated with a central germinal center made up of larger mononuclear cells. They appear within one week after the onset of acute *H. pylori* infection, and are uncommon in non-*H. pylori*-infected gastric mucosa. The number of lymphoid follicles correlates with the titer of serum IgG anti-*H. pylori* antibodies. Lymphoid follicles accompanying *H.pylori* gastritis are involved in the genesis of primary gastric lymphoma. The pathogenesis may involve stimulation of B cells with the ability for unsuppressed proliferation by activated T cells within the follicles (Egan et al).

H. pylori-associated chronic gastritis progresses with two main topographic patterns that have different clinical outcomes. The first pattern is antral predominant gastritis, characterized by inflammation mostly limited to the antrum and typical of individuals who develop duodenal ulcers. The second pattern is one of progressive pan-gastritis or multifocal atrophic gastritis, characterized by active infection of both the gastric corpus and antrum with progressive development of gastric atrophy and intestinal metaplasia. *H. pylori*-infected individuals who develop gastric carcinom and gastric ulcers usually show this pattern of gastritis.

Atrophic gastritis *H. pylori* infection can increase or decrease gastric acid secretion or exert no effect on the level of secretion. The factors that predict the impact on acid secretion are the location and severity of the inflammation in the stomach and the dysregulation of the normal acid inhibitory mechanisms associated with the presence of the infection. Three pathways figure prominently in the stimulation of acid secretion by the gastric mucosa. These include:

1) acetylcholine, which is released by the vagus nerve

2) histamine, released locally by enterochromaffin-like cells and

3) gastrin, released by the gastric antrum and carried via blood circulation to act on ECL cells and parietal cells (Egan et al).

Normally, changes in gastric acidity in response to meals are dependent on a negative feedback mechanism where high pH and proteins in the meal stimulate antral G cells to produce gastrin, which in turn stimulates the parietal cells in the gastric corpus to secrete acid. As the buffering capacity of the meal is exhausted, intragastric pH falls and when it declines below pH 3, antral D cells are stimulated to secrete somatostatin, which down-regulates gastrin and histamine secretion and thus suppresses acid secretion . This inhibitory mechanism is disrupted by the presence of *H. pylori* infection, leading to constant stimulation of gastrin secretion, resulting in more acid being secreted for longer periods of time. The duodenal mucosa employs a number of mechanisms to protect it from acid injury. The mucosa is covered with a viscoelastic mucus gel layer that acts as a physical barrier to acid and also secretes bicarbonate, which neutralizes the effects of gastric acid. Gastric metaplasia of the duodenum can occur as a result of continued high acid exposure, and this metaplasia appears to be essential for *H. pylori* colonization of the duodenal mucosa. Gastric metaplasia occurs most commonly in the first part of the duodenum corresponding to the most common site of duodenal ulcers. Gastric atrophy, gastric ulcer, and gastric cancer are associated with pan-gastritis, multifocal atrophy, and hyposecretion of acid. The development of pan-gastritis and multifocal atrophy is determined by a number of host and bacterial factors that favor the development of pan-gastritis over antral predominant gastritis. Although *H. pylori* is more tolerant of a low pH than most bacteria, it cannot proliferate as effectively in areas of higher acid production such as the gastric corpus. Conversely, a low acid output may allow the spread of *H. pylori* infection within the stomach with resultant inflammation of the gastric corpus. When inflammation affects the gastric corpus, parietal cells are inhibited, leading to reduced acid secretion that becomes permanent when corpus atrophy develops; this atrophy is characterized by the loss of oxyntic cells and the development of intestinal metaplasia.

Pepsinogen is a precursor for pepsin, a digestive enzyme specifically produced in the gastric mucosa. The human stomach expresses two isozymogens, pepsinogen 1 (PG1) and pepsinogen 2 (PG2), with different biochemical and immunological properties. Although PG1 is produced by chief and mucous neck cells, PG2 is produced not only by these cells, but also by cardiac, pyloric, and duodenal Brunner gland cells. The distribution of PG2-producing cells is thus widespread throughout the entire stomach. As gastric atrophy develops, chief cells are replaced by pyloric glands resulting in a decrease in PG1 whereas the decrease in PG2 is minimal. Therefore, both low serum PG1 and a low PG1/PG2 ratio are serologic markers of gastric atrophy. These markers, in combination with *H. pylori* antibody can identify patients at risk of gastric cancer development. Gastrin peptides are mainly synthesized in antroduodenal G cells, from which they are released into the blood to regulate gastric acid secretion and mucosal growth The major gastrin forms in tissue and plasma are gastrin-34 and gastrin-17, but gastrin-71, gastrin-14, and gastrin-6 have also been identified. Gastrin- 17 is a major form of gastrin peptides and is found in tissue and serum. It is dependent on intragastric acidity but also on the number of G cells in the antral mucosa. Gastrin-17 decreases along with an increasing grade of atrophic antral gastritis as G cells are lost. In atrophic gastritis involving the corpus alone there is a reduction in intragastric acidity, which stimulates the release of gastrin from antral G cells. Using both pepsinogen and gastrin-17 as markers, it may be possible to identify the pattern of gastritis by serologic testing when gastritis is limited to the corpus. Gastrin-17 levels may be high, whereas PG1 or the PG1/PG2 ratio is low (Weck et al).

Metaplastic atrophic gastritis does not cause symptoms and is often found incidentally on biopsy of the stomach in patients undergoing upper endoscopy. However, intestinal metaplasia is associated with gastric achlorhydria, which may result in small intestinal bacterial overgrowth with symptoms of bloating, flatulence, abdominal discomfort and diarrhea.

Metaplastic atrophic gastritis have two main subtypes, autoimmune and environmental metaplastic atrophic gastritis (AMAG and EMAG).

Autoimmune metaplastic atrophic gastritis (AMAG) is an inherited form of metaplastic atrophic gastritis that is associated with an immune response in the oxyntic mucosa directed against parietal cells and intrinsic factor. The chronic inflammation, gland atrophy, and epithelial metaplasia of AMAG are closely paralleled by elevated serum antibodies to parietal cells and to intrinsic factor, reflecting its autoimmune origin. The immune-mediated loss of parietal cell mass leads to both profound hypochlorhydria and inadequate production of intrinsic factor, which leads to vitamin B12 malabsorption and pernicious anemia.

Pacients with AMAG also may present hypergastrinemia as a result of uninhibited gastrin secretion due to parietal cell loss and achlorhydria, decreased serum pepsinogen I due to loss of zymogenic chief cells in the oxyntic mucosa, iron deficiency anemia due to hypochlorhydria. Under normal circumstances, gastric acid enhances iron absorption, by converting the ferric form of iron into the more absorbable ferrous form and by peptic denaturing the proteins bound to dietary iron.

Hypochlorhydria in AMAG decreases bioavailable iron, leading to iron deficiency.

Environmental metaplastic atrophic gastritis (EMAG) is due to the effects of H. pylori infection on the gastric mucosa. Unlike AMAG, mucosal changes in patients with EMAG affect both the corpus and antrum in a multifocal distribution, but with heaviest involvement of the antrum. In addition, EMAG differs from AMAG in a number of other ways: gastric acid production does not disappear entirely, serum gastrin is not elevated, parietal cell and intrinsic factor autoantibodies and pernicious anemia are absent. There is a higher risk for gastric ulcer compared with AMAG, presumably due to the protective effect of the accompanying hypochlorhydria in the latter disorder. Patients with EMAG are at increased risk for gastric cancer, particularly the intestinal type.

MALT limphoma. Gastric MALT lymphoma is a rare type of non-Hodgkin lymphoma that is characterized by the slow multiplication of B lymphocytes, a type of immune cell, in the stomach lining. This cancer represents approximately 12 percent of the extranodal(outside of lymph nodes) non-Hodgkin lymphoma that occurs among men and approximately 18 percent of extranodal non-Hodgkin lymphoma among women. Normally, the lining of the stomach lacks lymphoid (immune system) tissue, but development of this tissue is often stimulated in response to colonization of the lining by *H. pylori.*

Only in rare cases does this tissue give rise to MALT lymphoma. However, nearly all patients with gastric MALT lymphoma show signs of *H. pylori* infection, and the risk of developing this tumor is more than six times higher in infected people than in uninfected people. Eradication of *H. pylori* is the first choice in treating localized stage I gastric MALT lymphoma with *H. pylori* infection.

Duodenal Ulcer. *H. pylori* is present in more than 95% of patients with duodenal ulcers and in more than 80% of patients with gastric ulcer (Walsh and Peterson, 1995). The most convicing evidence for a causal relationship between *H. pylori* and PUD is healing of the ulcer following antibiotic therapy (Forbes et al., 1994; Graham et al., 1992; Hentschel et al., 1993). Patients with *H. pylori*-related duodenal ulcers have significantly higher basal and maximal acid output (El-Omar et al., 1995). Hyperchlorhydria promotes development of gastric metaplasia. The appearence of gastric epithelial cells in the duodenum allows colonization by *H. pylori*, which will establish a chronic inflammatory response, duodenitis (Khlulusi et al., 1996). The inflammation process and bacterial effect on the epithelial cells render the duodenal mucosa sensitive to gastric acidity, thus predisposing it to ulceration (McColl et al., 1998; Dixon, 2001; Atherton, 2006). In Western countries, duodenal ulcers are approximately fourfold more common than gastric ulcers; elsewhere, gastric ulcers are more common. Duodenal ulcers in particular occur between 20 and 50 years of age, while gastric ulcers predominantly arise in subjects over 40 years old (Kusters et al., 2006).

Gastric ulcer. Gastric ulcers mostly occur along the lesser curvature of the stomach, in particular, at the transition from corpus to antrum mucosa (Kusters et al., 2006). Gastric ulcers in contrast to duodenal ulcers, are associated with low acid secretion in addition to *H. pylori* infection (McColl et al., 1998; El-Omar et al., 1994). Colonization by *H. pylori* leads to continuing inflammatory cell infiltration, epithelial degeneration and increased exfoliation of epithelial cells. This leads to impaired mucin and bicarbonate production which comprises the mucus barrier and makes the tissue more susceptible to ulceration. Eradication of the *H. pylori* infection is associated with the cure of gastric ulcers.

Gastric adenocarcinoma. Gastric cancer is a major public health burden; globally, it is the fourth most common cancer. The incidence of gastric cancer varies throughout the world. High-risk areas include East Asian countries such as China, Japan and Korea, where the age-standardized incidence rate (ASR) is greater than 20 per 100 000. Intermediate risk countries (ASR 11–19/100 000) include Malaysia, Singapore and Taiwan, while low-risk areas (ASR < 10/100 000) include countries such as Australia, New Zealand, India and Thailand (Parkin et al., 2005).

Gastric cancer carcinogenesis is a multifactorial process, related to an interaction of host factors, *H. pylori* infection and environmental factors such as diet. There is a precancerous cascade, in which the gastric mucosa undergoes a series of changes resulting in gastritis, atrophy, intestinal metaplasia, and dysplasia, before developing eventually into gastric cancer (Correa et al., 2004). Epidemiological studies in humans and experimental infections in rodents have clearly demonstrated that sustained interactions between *H. pylori* and its host significantly increase the risk for atrophic gastritis, intestinal metaplasia, and distal gastric adenocarcinoma, and colonization by *H. pylori* is the strongest identified risk factor for malignancies that arise within the stomach (reviewed in Peek & Blaser, 2002). In 1994, the World Health Organization (WHO) and the International Agency for Research on Cancer (IARC) classified *H. pylori* as a carcinogen (IARC, 1994).

Gastric cancer occurs as a net result of long-term gastric mucosal infection with *H. pylori* and chronic inflammation. Gastritis that involves the acid-secreting corpus region results in hypochlorhydria, progressive gastric atrophy, and an increased risk of gastric cancer. The reports show that hypochlorhydric patients have less dense *H. pylori* colonization, body-predominant colonization and gastritis, and increase prevalence of body atrophy and intestinal metaplasia (El-Omar et al., 1997).

The difference in prevalence of infection versus incidence in gastric cancer (approx. 1%) suggests multifactorial etiology – such as differences in bacterial strains, host genotypes, and environmental

53

conditions (reviewed in Peek & Blaser, 2002). Due to the high prevalence of *H. pylori* infection, however, gastric adenocarcinoma is one of the most common cancers in the world and it is the second leading cause of cancer-related deaths, with almost 800.000 new diagnoses and 630.000 deaths per year. In particular, strains that carry the *cag* pathogenicity island and the *vacA* gene, i.e. the more virulent Type I strains, are significantly associated with overt disease (Gerhard *et al.*, 1999; Prinz *et al.*, 2001; Xiang *et al.*, 1995). Uang *et al.* conducted a meta-analysis to estimate the magnitude of the risk for gastric cancer associated with *cagA* seropositivity. *H. pylori* and *cagA* seropositivity significantly increased the risk for gastric cancer by 2.3- and 2.9-fold, respectively. Among *H. pylori*-infected populations, infection with *cagA* positive strains further increased the risk for gastric cancer 1.6-fold (95% CI: 1.2–2.2) overall and 2.0-fold (95% CI: 1.2–3.3) for non-cardia gastric cancer.

Although *H. pylori* components clearly influence disease risk, they are not absolute determinants of carcinogenesis, which has highlighted the need to identify host factors that also contribute to the development of gastric cancer. Individual differences in host responses are of major importance and polymorphism of IL-1β (pro-inflammatory cytokine with potent acid-suppressive properties) is the first the host risk factor for *H. pylori* associated gastric cancer. Polymorphisms within the human *IL-1* ß gene promoter that are associated with increased expression of

54

IL-1ß, heighten the risk for gastric adenocarcinoma (El-Omar et al., 2000). In addition to IL-1β, TNF-α is a proinflammatory acid-suppressive cytokine that is increased within *H. pylori*-colonized human gastric mucosa. Polymorphisms that increase TNF-α expression, as well as low-expression polymorphisms within the locus controlling expression of the anti-inflammatory cytokine IL-10 are associated with an enhanced risk of gastric cancer. The combinatorial effect of IL-1β, TNF-α, and IL-10 polymorphisms on the development of cancer has also been determined, and risk increases progressively with an increasing number of proinflammatory polymorphisms, to the point that three high-risk polymorphisms increase the risk of cancer 27-fold over baseline (El-Omar et al., 2003).

Extragastric manifestations of H. Pylori infection. Helicobacter pylori infection has been reported in the association with several extragastric diseases like:

- hematologic disorders such as iron-deficiency anemia and idiopathic thrombocytopenic purpura,
- vascular disorders such as ischemic heart disease, cerebral stroke, primary Raynaud phenomenon and primary headache,
- autoimmune diseases such as Sjogren's syndrome, Henoch-Schonlein purpura, autoimmune thyroiditis,
- idiopathic arrythmias,
- Parkinson's disease,

- non arterial anterior optic ischemic neuropathy,
- cutaneous disorders, such as rosacea,
- pediatric diseases such as growth retardation and sudden infant death syndrome,
- renal failure,
- diabetes mellitus,
- respiratory disorders and glaucoma,

The evidence of data about these extragastric manifestations of H. Pylori infection has not been complete and is not widely known.

Increasing evidence supports H. Pylori infection as a cause of iron deficiency anemia, while moderate evidence sustains H. Pylori infection as a cause of idiophatic trombocytopenic purpura (Triantafillidis et al 2006).

Several theories try to explain the possible mechanisms for iron deficiency anemia. These include: in H. Pylori subjects with positive gastritis concomitent changes in intragastric pH and ascorbic acid are present leading to impairment of iron absorbtion. Also H. Pylori can act as sequestering factor for lactoferrin. These models, however, don't explain why all infected individuals do not suffer from iron deficiency anemia.

The role of *H. pylori* in the pathogenesis of ITP was first described by Gasbarrini *et al.* The possible mechanism would be that H. Pylori infection can induce antibody production in response to antigens that cross-react against various platelet glycoprotein antigens. The platelet count in patients with ITP returns to normal levels after *H. pylori* eradication. Improvement in platelet count after eradication therapy is obtained as well in adults as in children. The platelet recovery is a result of the eradication therapy and the eradication of the bacteria is partly explained by the reduction in autoantibody production. Thus, *H. pylori* assessment should be performed in chronic ITP patients and eradication therapy should be attempted in positive test cases.

9. Diagnostic methods

Diagnostic tests for *H. pylori* are generally divided into two categories: invasive and noninvasive. Invasive tests comprise the histological examination of gastric specimens.

Noninvasive tests are based on peripheral samples such as blood, breath, stools, urine, and saliva, in order to detect antibodies, bacterial antigens, or urease activity. The choice of a specific test always depends on local experience and clinical settings, but usually a combination of two methods is often recommended since, for example, the detection of *H. pylori*-specific antibodies does not ultimately reflect a current infection (Bauer and Meyer, 2011).

Performing endoscopy solely to diagnosis *H. pylori* infection is not appropriate; there are three methods—biopsy urease test, histology, and (less often) culture—to identify the organism during an otherwise indicated endoscopic procedure (Sleissenger et al).

The American Gastroenterological Association has recommended that an upper endoscopy be performed in patients who are older than 45 years with new-onset dyspepsia and in patients younger than 55 years who have "alarm" symptoms (weight loss, recurrent vomiting, dysphagia, evidence of bleeding, anemia). Dyspeptic patients in whom an empirical trial of proton pump inhibitors and eradication of *H. pylori* do not relieve symptoms should undergo prompt endoscopic evaluation as well. The basis for these recommendations is the low incidence of gastric cancer in individuals younger than 45 years. Early endoscopy is also recommended in patients younger than 45 years who have a family history of gastric cancer, emigrated from a country with a high rate of gastric cancer, or had a prior partial gastrectomy.

Antral biopsies can be tested for urease activity using rapid ureas kits. One of the most widely used is the CLOtest (Campylobacter-Like Organism, Ballard Medical, Draper, UT). With this technique, one or two pieces of tissue are placed in an agar well that contains urea and a pH reagent. Urease cleaves urea to liberate ammonia, producing an alkaline pH and a resultant color change. The CLOtest may become positive as early as one hour after collection, but a final reading at 24 hours is recommended.

The sensitivity of biopsy urease tests is approximately 90 to 95 percent, and specificity is 95 to 100 percent. False positive tests are unusual. However, false negative results can appear in patients with active gastrointestinal bleeding or with the use of PPIs, H2 antagonists, antibiotics, or bismuth-containing compounds. Same problem occur in urea breath test and fecal antigen test because these drugs decrease the bacteria density. Thus, to the patients with these conditions stopping PPIs or antibiotics at least 2 weeks prior to endoscopy is indicated.Other alterative would be to perform serology test which is not influenced by current treatment.

Routine culture for H. pylori is not currently recommended. Culture is only indicated for resistant cases to at least 2 cycles of therapy. Antibiotic sensitivity tests are recommended in these situations.

Noninvasive tests for the diagnosis of H. pylori include urea breath testing (UBT), stool antigen testing and serology. Urea breath testing is based upon the hydrolysis of urea by H. pylori to produce CO_2 and ammonia. A labeled carbon isotope is given by mouth; H. pylori liberate tagged CO_2 that can be detected in breath samples. The sensitivity and specificity of UBT are approximately 88 to 95 percent and 95 to 100 percent. False negative results have the same limitations like rapid urease test.

Guidelines recommend that serologic testing should be used especially in high prevalence populations. Treatment is indicated to patients without prior treatments for H. pylori. If the patient had a history of H. pylori treatment, antibiotic exposure for other infection or is from a low prevalence population, secondary testing with a stool or breath test to confirm the initial result is appropriate. Confirmation of eradication of H. pylori infection using serology test (decrease of Ig G titre) should be used after at least one year or more following treatment. This is rarely done except in settings where a patient cannot discontinue antisecretory therapies.

The stool antigen assay is also useful for documenting eradication after at least 4 weeks following treatment.

10. Current therapies and antibiotic resistance rates

The pathogenicity of this microorganism is regarded by some as equivocal and therefore it is still controversial if the eradication would be the best approach. The controversy centers is around on whether to eliminate the organism in all infected individuals, or only in symptomatic patients on the grounds that the microorganism may be a commensal and provide benefits to the a asymptomatic infected person. "Treaters" suggest that eradication of the microorganism would likely reduce the development of gastric inflammation, development of peptic ulcer disease (especially in those patients who are also taking non-steroidal anti-inflammatory drugs, and with the theoretical benefit of reducing the progression to gastric malignancy). "Commensalists" suggest that *H. pylori*, rather than being a pathogen, is in fact a commensal, and its eradication would worsens gastro-esophageal reflux disease or even induces asthma. However, while clear that the inhabitants of the lower gut do not cause inflammation and hence can be regarded as commensals, in the case of *H. pylori*, gastritis is inevitable associated with an intense immune response, not characteristics of symbionts (Sachs and Scott, 2012).

According to the Maastricht IV consensus treatment of Helicobacter pylori should be indicated for (Malfertheiner et al, 2012):

- patients with gastroduodenal diseases such as peptic ulcer disease and low grade gastric, mucosa associated lymphoid tissue (MALT) lymphoma;
- univestigated dyspepia-test and treat strategy for patients under age of 45
- patients with atrophic gastritis;
- first degree relatives of patients with gastric cancer;
- patients with unexplained iron deficiency anaemia;
- patients with chronic idiopathic thrombocytopenic purpura.

Also, for prevention of gastric cancer, eradication of Helicobacter pylori should be done for high risk patients:

- first degree relatives of the family members of patients with gastric cancer
- patients treated by endoscopic resection or partial surgical resection
- patients with cancer risk: severe pangastritis, corporeal gastritis
- severe atrophy
- patients with PPI treatment longer than one year
- patients with strong environmental factors for gastric cancers: heavy smoking, high exposure to coal, dust, cement, quartz, workers in quarries
- H. pylori positive cancer with a fear of gastric cancer

The test-and-treat strategy for H. pylori infection is a proven management strategy for patients with uninvestigated dyspepsia who are under the age of 45 yr and have no "alarm features" (bleeding, anemia, early satiety, unexplained weight loss, progressive dysphagia, odynophagia, recurrent vomiting, family history of GI cancer, previous esophagogastric malignancy).

For the patients with alarm features or with the age after 45, upper GI endoscopy is mandatory and Helicobacter pylori can be tested during this investigation by rapid urease test or biopsy.

Confirmation of eradication should be performed in patients (Chey and Wong, 2007):

- who receive treatment of *H. pylori* for peptic ulcer disease,
- with persistent dyspeptic symptoms despite the test-and-treat strategy
- with *H. pylori*-associated MALT lymphoma and
- who have undergone resection of early gastric cancer.
- Cag A positive patients (recommendation added as result of authors study)

The choosen method for eradication confirmation is by urea respiratory breath test, fecal antigen or rapid urease test when endoscopy is neded. It should be performed at least 4 weeks after treatment completion, otherwise is a risk of false negative test. Antibody tests should be avoided posttreatment because they remain positive prolonged periods of time.

Recent studies suggest that eradication rates achieved by first-line treatment with a proton pump inhibitor (PPI), clarithromycin, and amoxicillin have decreased to 70–85%, in part due to increasing clarithromycin resistance.

Nonetheless the importance of *H pylori* infection and virulence factors cannot be dismissed. There is no doubt that the eradication of *H pylori* infection leads to healing of duodenal ulceration and the risk of recurrence is greatly reduced. There is also no doubt about the strong association of *H pylori* and virulence factors with duodenal ulceration in countries where the overall prevalence of *H pylori* infection is relatively low (Tovey et al., 2006).

Eradication therapy for *H. pylori* was unknown prior to 1984. Earliest attempts at treating the infection were carried out by Barry Marshall using monotherapy and later dual therapy. Subsequent developments focused upon finding appropriate available antimicrobial agents in various combinations. Triple Therapy comprising of a proton pump inhibitor (PPI), amoxicillin, and clarithromycin (standard triple therapies), given for a week has been recommended as the treatment of choice at several consensus conferences, yielded high efficacy, providing eradication rates comparable to those expected for other prevalent bacterial infections. Other treatments have also been proposed, including metronidazole, tetracycline, fluoroquinolones, and rifampycins. Unfortunately, in successive years the effectiveness of many of the frequently recommended *H. pylori* infection treatment regimens has been increasingly compromised by antimicrobial resistance (Rimbara et al., 2011).

Establishing the optimal drug therapy depends to a large extent on antimicrobial concentrations in the stomach, an environment that is not easily accessible to some medications. The first hurdle for bioavailability of antibiotics is the acidity of the gastric lumen (pH 1.4). For example clarithromycin, is degraded in the lumen mainly through the action of acid and pepsin. The co-administration of gastric acidity inhibitors has been shown to significantly reduce eradication failure. For antibiotics such as tetracycline, clarithromycin and amoxicillin, bacterial growth is essential for their efficacy. The average intra gastric pH achieved by proton pump inhibitors is ~ 4.0, still low enough for many of the microorganisms to multiply. More effective inhibition of acid secretion would likely improve eradication by the use of a bactericidal drug such as amoxicillin, to which current resistance is < 1%. This would result in dual therapy with BID (twice daily) administration of the inhibitor of acid secretion and amoxicillin (Sachs and Scott, 2012). The second hurdle is represented by the gastric mucus. To successfully kill the bacteria present in the stomach it is necessary that the drug is delivered to the entire surface of the stomach and penetrates across the mucus layer from gastric lumen to epithelial surface (or vice versa) (Wu et al., 2012).

Conventional triple therapies for *H. pylori* eradication have recently shown a disappointing reduction in effectiveness in many countries. The main reason for failure was found to be the bacterial resistance which varies in different geographic areas, and it has been correlated with the consumption of antibiotics in the general population (Megraud, 2004). Another important factor is polymorphism of the CYP2C19 isoenzyme that is responsible for the biotransformation of several PPIs: significant differences in eradication rates have been observed between homozygous and heterozygous extensive metabolizers and poor metabolizers of PPIs (omeprazole being the most affected followed by lansoprazole). As a consequence, the use of higher doses may be required (Gasparetto et al., 2012).

Standard triple therapy which represents the accepted standard therapy for *H. pylori* is known to be susceptible to clarithromycin, and local antimicrobial resistance rates are below to 20% (Malfertheiner et al., 2007). Newer treatment regimens: sequential, quadruple, concomitant, and hybrid therapies and various combinations of new and old antibiotics aimed at eradicating the organism more effectively are increasing in popularity (Basu et al., 2011; Hsu et al., 2008). A combination of a PPI, amoxicillin and levofloxacin, as first-line regimen, has been associated with favorable results, with mean eradication rates of about 90% (Rispo *et al.* 2007; Gisbert et al. 2007; Antos *et al.* 2006; Lee *et al.* 2006; Marzio *et al.* 2006; Di Caro *et al.* 2002; Cammarota *et al.* 2000). It has been suggested that levofloxacin-based therapies may also represent an alternative when two (or more) consecutive eradication treatments have failed to eradicate the infection (Liou et al., 2010).

After failure of a combination of PPI, amoxicillin and clarithromycin, a theoretically correct alternative would be the use, as second option, of other PPI-based triple therapy including amoxicillin (that does not induce resistance) and metronidazole (an antibiotic not used in the first trial), and several authors have reported encouraging results with this strategy (Ueki *et al.* 2009; Murakami *et al.* 2008, 2006; Shirai *et al.* 2007; Matsuhisa *et al.* 2006; Nagahara *et al.* 2004; Shimoyama *et al.* 2004; Isomoto *et al.* 2003; Miwa *et al.* 2003). Another alternative, the use of a quadruple regimen (i.e. PPI, bismuth, tetracycline and metronidazole), has been generally used as the optimal second-line therapy after PPI-clarithromycin-amoxicillin failure, and has been the recommended 'rescue' regimen in several guidelines (Malfertheiner *et al.* 2007; Gisbert *et al.* 2000; Lam and Talley, 1998).

A systematic review of studies concerning primary *H. pylori* antibiotic resistance performed by De Francesco et al. (2010) showed that worldwide *H. pylori* antibiotic resistance towards different antibiotics is increasing. *H. pylori* antibiotic resistance rates all over the world are 17.2% for clarithromycin, 26.7% for metronidazole, 11.2% for amoxicillin, and 16.2% for levofloxacin.

Clarithromycin remains the most powerful antibiotic against *H. pylori* currently available and primary resistance towards this drug has been found to be the main factor hampering the efficacy of standard therapies (Magraud, 2004). In Europe, a marked difference has been observed between Southern and Northern Europe. Higher resistance rates of clarithromycin in adults are observed in southern European countries (from 23.5% in Spain to 40.3% in the United Kingdom), America (from 21.6% in the United States to 76.3% in Mexico) and Asia (from 9%-12% in Japan to 41.9% in Korea). The prevalence of antibiotic resistance in various regions is correlated with the widespread use of antibiotics for upper respiratory tract infections in the region, while in countries with a prudent consumption of macrolides continues to be low (Giorgio et al., 2013).

Various polymerase chain reaction-based studies have demonstrated that point mutations in the peptidyl transferase region, encoded in domain V of 23S rRNA, are responsible of *H. pylori* resistance towards clarithromycin. The more frequent mutations associated with clarithromycin resistance are the adenine to transitions at positions 2142 and 2143 of rRNA (A2143G and A2143C).

The overall European metronidazole resistance is 17% being constantly less that 40% in all countries, but a significantly lower prevalence in Central and Eastern parts, whilst it is distinctly higher in both Asia and America. As for clarithromycin, reports demonstrated a significantly higher prevalence of metronidazole resistance in females. The current European guidelines on *H. pylori* management suggest that first-line therapy should be tailored according to both clarithromycin and metronidazole resistance (De Francesco et al., 2010). Regarding the mechanism of metronidazole resistance in *H. pylori*, complex and multiple mechanisms are implicated, including point mutations, deletion in *rdxA* gene, which encode an oxygen-insensitive NADPH nitroreductase and pump efflux system.

The prevalence of levofloxacin resistance seems to be increasing worldwide; therefore its use should be reserved as a second-line therapy. Point mutations in the Quinolones Resistance-Determining Region of *gyrA* prevent binding between the antibiotic and the enzyme, conferring antibiotic bacterial resistance to quinolones (De Francesco et al., 2012).

Resistance rates towards either tetracycline or amoxicillin remain particularly low or absent in all regions except Africa, where the prevalence of tetracycline resistance is 43.9% (Magraud, 2004), most likely this is due to the requirement to develop simultaneous mutations in the respective genes.

Primary *H. pylori* resistance towards antibiotics involved in the current eradication regimens affects the therapeutic outcome. Given the described geographical variability, the development of better treatments for *H. pylori* infection should take into consideration the distribution of antibiotic resistance among affected populations in different geographical areas (Gasparetto et al., 2012). On this basis constant surveillance of antibiotic resistance rates is meaningful for *H. pylori* infection management in clinical practice (De Francesco et al, 2010). Moreover eradication of infection should always be confirmed after treatment in order to provide feedback regarding local effectiveness and an early warning of increasing resistance (Rimbara et al., 2011).

It is important to perform culture and standard susceptibility testing to antimicrobial agents in a region or population of high clarithromycin resistance before prescription of the first-line treatment if the standard clarithromycin-containing triple therapy is being considered. Furthermore, culture and standard susceptibility testing should be considered in all regions before second-line treatment if endoscopy is carried out for another reason and generally when a second-line treatment has failed.

Following the European Medicines Agency recommendation on evaluation of medicinal products indicated for treatment of bacterial infection, three categories of bacterial species can be defined according to their susceptibility to a given antibiotic: usually susceptible (0-10% resistant), inconstantly susceptible (10-50% resistant) and usually resistant (>50% resistant). H pylori now falls into the second category, except for Northern Europe

In order to take into account the CIs of the prevalence obtained and the regional differences in a given country, a threshold of 15-20% was recommended to separate the regions of high and low clarithromycin resistance (figure 1).

In areas of low clarithromycin resistance, clarithromycin-containing treatments are recommended for first-line empirical treatment; Bismuth-containing quadruple therapy is also an alternative. Extending the duration of PPI-clarithromycin-containing triple therapies from 7 to 10-14 days improves the eradication success by about 5% and may be considered. After failure of a PPI clarithromycin-containing treatment, either a bismuth-containing quadruple therapy or levofloxacin-containing triple therapy is recommended.

In areas of high clarithromycin resistance, bismuth-containing quadruple therapies are recommended for first-line empirical treatment. If this regimen is not available, sequential treatment or a non-bismuth quadruple therapy is recommended. After failure of bismuth containing quadruple therapy, levofloxacin containing triple therapy is recommended (Malfertheiner et al., 2012).

After failure of second-line therapy, treatment should be guided by antimicrobial susceptibility testing, whenever possible.

In the study of Ilie et al. in 2011, on Helicobacter pylori cultivation from gastric biopsies on 226 patients, the resistance rates for the antibiotics used in the classic triple therapy proved to be high, i.e. 85% for metronidazole, 40% for amoxicillin and 26% for clarithromycin. The isolated strains proved to be sensitive to ciprofloxacin and levofloxacin.

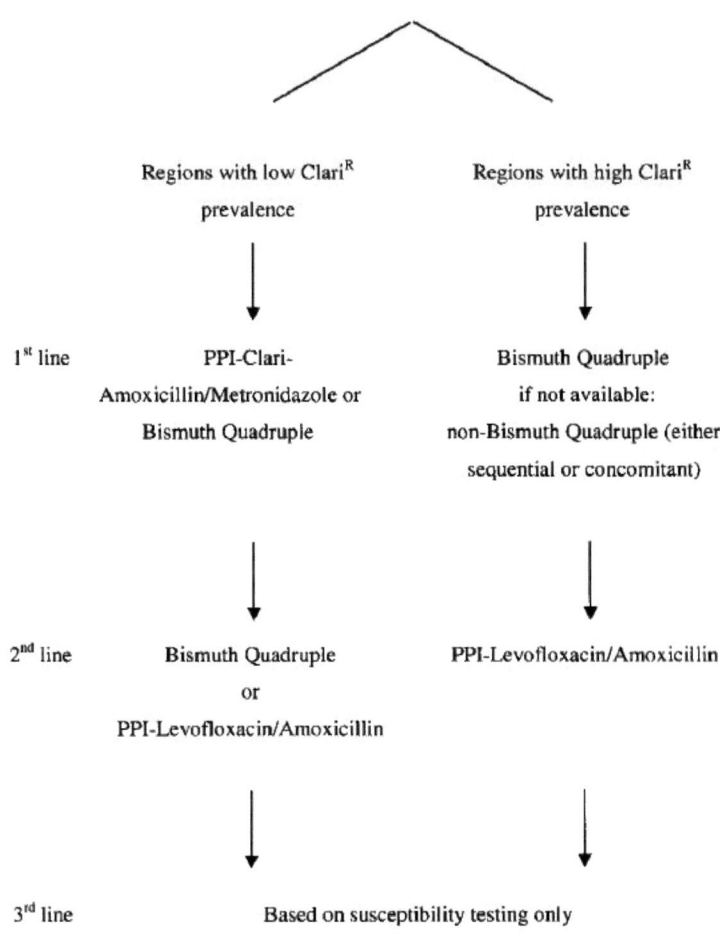

Figure 6- Treatment according to Clarithromicin resistance (from Maastricht IV Consensus Report)

11. Conclusions

Helicobacter pylori infection represents a public health problem, especially in eastern European countries.

Cag A strains are virulent, being associated with resistance to first line therapy, bleeding gastroduodenal ulcer, gastric polyps and gastric cancer.

An important percent of bleeding gastroduodenal ulcers cag A positive were also NSAID (non-steroidal anti-inflammatory drugs), proving that in NSAID ulcers, H. pylori must also be tested, the sum of cag A positivity and NSAID presence, increasing the risk of haemorrhage.

The highest titers of cag A antibodies (more than 100 arbU/ml) in the study realised by Ilie et al in 2011, was found for resistance to first line therapy, bleeding gastroduodenal ulcers, NSAID negative and gastric cancer.

Following these results we can add to the Helicobacter pylori treatment recommendations also the presence of cag A Ig G antibodies concomitant with active infection (rapid urease test positive or breath test or fecal antigen for H. pylori).

Also, knowing the increased rate of resistance to first line therapy of cag A positive patients, we recommend verification of H. pylori eradication by fecal antigen or urea breath test, one month after completing the treatment.

At patients cag A positive with active infection we can start treatment with Bismuth quadruple therapy or directly with Levofloxacin, Amoxicillin and PPI in order to avoid resistance to first line therapy.

References

1. Makola, Diklar MB ChB, PhD; Peura, David A. MD; Crowe, Sheila E. MD. Helicobacter pylori Infection and Related Gastrointestinal Diseases. *Journal of Clinical Gastroenterology*: July 2007 - Volume 41 - Issue 6 - pp 548-558 doi: 10.1097/MCG.0b013e318030e3c3 Alimentary Tract: Clinical Reviews

2. González Carolina - Romo, Salama Nina R, Burgeño-Ferreira Juan, Differences in Genome Content among Helicobacter pylori Isolates from Patients with Gastritis, Duodenal Ulcer or Gastric Cancer Reveal Novel Disease-*Associated Genes Infect Immun*. 2009 May; 77(5): 2201–2211. 10.1128/IAI.01284-08 PMCID: PMC2681767

3. Backert, S., T. Schwarz, S. Miehlke, C. Kirsch, C. Sommer, T. Kwok, M. Gerhard, U. Goebel, N. Lehn, W. Koenig, and T. F. Meyer. 2004. Functional analysis of the *cag* pathogenicity island in *Helicobacter pylori* isolates from patients with gastritis, peptic ulcer, and gastric cancer. *Infect. Immun.* 721043-1056. [PMC free article] [PubMed]

4. Peek, R. M., Jr., G. G. Miller, K. T. Tham, G. I. Perez-Perez, X. Zhao, J. C. Atherton, and M. J. Blaser. 1995. Heightened inflammatory response and cytokine expression in vivo to *cagA+ Helicobacter pylori* strains. *Lab. Investig.* 73760-770. [PubMed]

5. Weel, J. F., R. W. van der Hulst, Y. Gerrits, P. Roorda, M. Feller, J. Dankert, G. N. Tytgat, and A. van der Ende. 1996. The interrelationship between cytotoxin-associated gene A, vacuolating cytotoxin, and *Helicobacter pylori*-related diseases. *J. Infect. Dis.* 1731171-1175. [PubMed]

6. Hunt, R. H. 1996. The role of *Helicobacter pylori* in pathogenesis: the spectrum of clinical outcomes. *Scand. J. Gastroenterol.* 31(Suppl. 220):3–9.

7. Atherton John C. and Blaser Martin. Coadaptation of Helicobacter pylori and humans: ancient history, modern implications. *The Journal of*

Clinical Investigation http://www.jci.org Volume 119 Number 9 September 2009; 2475-2487.

8. Banatvala, N., et al. 1993. The cohort effect and Helicobacter pylori. *J. Infect. Dis.* 168:219–221.

9. Chen, Y., and Blaser, M.J. 2008. Helicobacter pylori colonization is inversely associated with childhood asthma. *J. Infect. Dis.* 198:553–560.

10. McNamaraa D., El-Omar E.. Helicobacter pylori infection and the pathogenesis of gastric cancer: A paradigm for host–bacterial interactions. *Digestive and Liver Disease* 40 (2008) 504–509

11. Sachs, G., Weeks, D.L., Melchers, K., and Scott, D.R. 2003. The gastric biology of Helicobacter pylori. *Annu. Rev. Physiol.* 65:349–369.

12. Weeks, D.L., Eskandari, S., Scott, D.R., and Sachs, G. 2000. A H+-gated urea channel: the link between Helicobacter pylori urease and gastric colonization. *Science.* 287:482–485.

13. Parsonnett J. *H pylori*: the size of the problem. *Gut* 1998;43:S6–8.

14. Backhed, F., et al. 2003. Gastric mucosal recognition of Helicobacter pylori is independent of Toll like receptor 4. *J. Infect. Dis.* 187:829–836.

15. Lee, S.K., et al. 2003. Helicobacter pylori flagellins have very low intrinsic activity to stimulate human gastric epithelial cells via TLR5. *Microbes Infect.* 5:1345–1356.

16. Johannes G. Kusters, Arnoud H. M. van Vliet, and Ernst J. Kuipers. Pathogenesis of Helicobacter pylori Infection. *Clin Microbiol Rev.* 2006 July; 19(3): 449–490. doi: 10.1128/CMR.00054-05

17. Krasteva A, Panov V, Oral cavity and systemic diseases – H*elicobacter pylori* and dentistry, 2011, *Biotechnol. & Biotechnol.* Eq. 2011, **25**(3), 2447-2541

18. Seiji Shiota1,2, Rumiko Suzuki1, Yoshio Yamaoka1,3. The significance of virulence factors in Helicobacter pylori. *Journal of Digestive Diseases.* Volume 14, Issue 7, pages 341–349, July 2013

19. Hideaki Higashi*, Ryouhei Tsutsumi*, Akiko Fujita*, Shiho Yamazaki, Masahiro Asaka, Takeshi Azuma and Masanori Hatakeyama. Biological activity of the Helicobacter pylori virulence factor CagA is determined by variation in the tyrosine phosphorylation sites. *PNAS*, October 29, 2002, vol. 99, no. 22, 14428 –14433.

20. Censini, S., et al. 1996. Cag, a pathogenicity island of Helicobacter pylori, encodes type I-specific and disease-associated virulence factors. *Proc. Natl. Acad.* Sci. U. S. A. 93:14648–14653.

21. Tegtmeyer Nicole, Wessler Silja, and Backert Steffen, FEBS J. Author manuscript; available in PMC 2012 April 1. Published in final edited form as: FEBS J. 2011 April; 278(8): 1190–1202. Published online 2011 February 25. doi: 10.1111/j.1742-4658.2011.08035.x PMCID: PMC3070773 NIHMSID: NIHMS269592

22. Joyce, EA, Glibert JV, Eaton KA, Plaut A., and Wright A. 2001. Differential gene expression from two transcriptional units in the cag pathogenicity island of Helicobacter pylori. *Infect. Immnun.* 69, 4202-4209.

23. Amsterdam Van K., Van Vliet AH, Kusters JG, Feller M, Dankert J and vand der Ende A. 2003. Induced Helicobacter pylori vacuolating cytotoxin VacA expression after initial colonization of human gastric epithelial cells. *FEMS Immunol Med Microbiol.* 39, 251-256.

24. Boonjakuakul JK, Canfield DR and Solnick JV. 2005. Comparison of Helicobacter pylori virulence gene expression in vitro and in the Rhesus macaque. *Infect. Immun.* 73. 4895-4904.

25. Boonjakuakul JK, Syvanen M, Suryaprasad A, Bowlus CL, and Solnick JV. 2004. Transcription profile of Helicobacter pylori in the human stomach reflects its physiology in vivo. *J. Infect. Dis.* 190, 946-956.

26. Kim N, Amrcus EA, Wen Y, Weeks, DL, Scott DR, Jung HC, Song IS, and Sachs G. 2004. Genes of Helicobacter pylori regulated by attachment to AGS cells. *Infect. Immun.* 72. 2358-2368.

27. Gieseler S., Konig B, Konig W and Backert S., 2005. Strain specific expression profile of virulence genes in Helicobacter pylori during infection of gastric epithelial cells and granulocytes. *Microbes Infect.* 7, 437-447.

28. Scott DR, Marcus EA, Wen Y, Oh J. and Sachs G. 2007. Gene expression in vivo shows that Helicobacter pylori colonizes an acidic niche on gastric surface. *Proc. Natl. Acad Sci* USA. 104, 7235-7240.

29. Castillo AR, Woodruff AJ, Connolly LE, Sause WE and Ottermann KM. 2008. Recombination based in vivo expression technology identifies Helicobacter pylori genes important for host colonization. *Infect. Immun.* 76. 5632-5644.

30. Hatakeyama M. Oncogenic mechanisms of the *Helicobacter pylori* CagA protein. *Nat Rev Cancer.* 2004;4:688–694.

31. Kwok, T., et al. 2007. Helicobacter exploits integrin for type IV secretion and kinase activation. *Nature.* 449:862–866.

32. Takagi J. Structural basis for ligand recognition by RGD (Arg-Gly-Asp)-dependent integrins. *Biochem Soc Trans.* 2004;32:403–406.

33. Backert S, Moese S, Selbach M, Brinkmann V, Meyer TF. Phosphorylation of tyrosine 972 of the *Helicobacter pylori* CagA protein is essential for induction of a scattering phenotype in gastric epithelial cells. *Mol Microbiol.* 2001;42:631–644.

34. Poppe M, Feller SM, Romer G, Wessler S. Phosphorylation of *Helicobacter pylori* CagA by c-Abl leads to cell motility. *Oncogene.* 2007;26:3462–3472.

35. Higashi, H., et al. 2002. Biological activity of the Helicobacter pylori virulence factor CagA is determined by variation in the tyrosine phosphorylation sites. *Proc. Natl. Acad.* Sci. U. S. A. 99:14428–14433.

36. Argent, R.H., et al. 2004. Determinants and consequences of different levels of CagA phosphorylation for clinical isolates of Helicobacter pylori. *Gastroenterology.* 127:514–523.

37. Yamaoka, Y., et al. 1999. Relationship between the cagA 3' repeat region of Helicobacter pylori, gastric histology, and susceptibility to low pH. *Gastroenterology*. 117:342–349.

38. Argent, R.H., Hale, J.L., El-Omar, E.M., and Atherton, J.C. 2008. Differences in Helicobacter pylori CagA tyrosine phosphorylation motif patterns between western and East Asian strains, and influences on interleukin-8 secretion. *J. Med. Microbiol*. 57:1062–1067.

39. Basso, D., et al. 2008. Clinical relevance of Helicobacter pylori cagA and vacA gene polymorphisms. *Gastroenterology*. 135:91–99.

40. Delahay, R.M., et al. 2008. The highly repetitive region of the Helicobacter pylori CagY protein comprises tandem arrays of an alpha-helical repeat module. *J. Mol. Biol*. **377**:956–971.

41. Seiji Shiota,1 Osamu Matsunari,1 Masahide Watada,1 and Yoshio Yamaoka1,2,† Serum Helicobacter pylori CagA antibody as a biomarker for gastric cancer in east-*Asian countries Future Microbiol*. 2010 December; 5(12): 1885–1893, doi: 10.2217/fmb.10.135.

42. Zhiyu Zhang, Qing Zheng, Xiaoyu Chen, Shudong Xiao, Wenzhong Liu and Hong Lu. The Helicobacter pylori duodenal ulcer promoting gene, dupA in China. *BMC Gastroenterology* 2008, 8:49 doi:10.1186/1471-230X-8-49

43. Lu, H., Hsu, P.I., Graham, D.Y., and Yamaoka, Y. 2005. Duodenal ulcer promoting gene of Helicobacter pylori. *Gastroenterology*. 128:833–848.

44. Gomes LI, Rocha GA, Rocha AM, Soares TF, Oliveira CA, Bittencourt PF, Queiroz DM: Lack of association between Helicobacter pylori infection with dupA-positive strains and gastroduodenal diseases in Brazilian patients. *Int J Med Microbiol* 2008, 298:223-30.

45. Argent RH, Burette A, Miendje Deyi VY, Atherton JC: The presence of dupA in Helicobacter pylori is not significantly associated with

duodenal ulceration in Belgium, South Africa, China, or North America. *Clin Infect Dis* 2007, 45:1204-6.

46. Chiarini, A., Cala, C., Bonura, C., Gullo, A., Giuliana, G., Peralta, S., D'Arpa, F. & Giammanco, A. (2008). Prevalence of virulence-associated genotypes of Helicobacter pylori and correlation with severity of gastric pathology in patients from western Sicily, Italy. *Eur J Clin Microbiol Infect Di*s 28, 437–446.

47. Dossumbekova, A., Prinz, C., Mages, J., Lang, R., Kusters, J. G., Van Vliet, A. H., Reindl, W., Backert, S., Saur, D. & other authors (2006).Helicobacter pylori HopH (OipA) and bacterial pathogenicity: geneticand functional genomic analysis of hopH gene polymorphisms. *J Infect. Dis* 194, 1346–1355.

48. Douraghi, M., Mohammadi, M., Oghalaie, A., Abdirad, A., Mohagheghi, M. A., Hosseini, M. E., Zeraati, H., Ghasemi, A., Esmaieli, M. & Mohajerani, N. (2008). dupA as a risk determinant in Helicobacter pylori infection. *J Med Microbiol* 57, 554–562.

49. Erzin, Y., Koksal, V., Altun, S., Dobrucali, A., Aslan, M., Erdamar, S., Dirican, A. & Kocazeybek, B. (2006). Prevalence of Helicobacter pylori vacA, cagA, cagE, iceA, babA2 genotypes and correlation with clinical outcome in Turkish patients with dyspepsia. *Helicobacter* 11, 574– 580.

50. Marshall, D. G., Dundon, W. S., Beesley, S. M. & Smyth, C. J. (1998). Helicobacter pylori – a conundrum of genetic diversity. *Microbiology* 144, 2925–2939.

51. Yamaoka, Y. (2008). Roles of the plasticity regions of Helicobacter pylori in gastroduodenal pathogenesis. *J Med Microbiol* 57, 545–553.

52. Hocker, M. & Hohenberger, P. (2003). *Helicobacter pylori* virulence factors – one part of a big picture. *Lancet* 362, 1231–1233.

53. Alvi, A., Devi, S. M., Ahmed, I., Hussain, M. A., Rizwan, M., Lamouliatte, H., Megraud, F. & Ahmed, N. (2007). Microevolution of

Helicobacter pylori type IV secretion systems in an ulcer disease patient over a ten-year period. *J Clin Microbiol* 45, 4039–4043.

54. Cover, T.L., Tummuru, M.K., Cao, P., Thompson, S.A., and Blaser, M.J. 1994. Divergence of genetic sequences for the vacuolating cytotoxin among Helicobacter pylori strains. *J. Biol. Chem.* 269:10566–10573.

55. Guadalupe Ayala, Julia Torres-Mena and Lizbeth Lopez-Carrillo. Association between Helicobacter pylori VacA antigens and gastric cancer depends on the detection method used: immunoblot versus neutralization of the vacuolating activity of VacA. *Journal of Medical Microbiology.* 2008. 57, 9-14.

56. Yoshio Yamaoka, Dong H. Kwon, and David Y. Graham. A Mr 34,000 proinflammatory outer membrane protein (oipA) of Helicobacter pylori. *PNAS* June 20, 2000 vol. 97 no. 13 7533–7538

57. Gerhard, M., et al. 1999. Clinical relevance of the Helicobacter pylori gene for blood-group antigen- binding adhesin. *Proc. Natl. Acad. Sci. U. S. A.* 96:12778–12783.

58. Odenbreit S, Swoboda K, Barwig I, Ruhl S, Borén T, Koletzko S, Haas R: Outer membrane protein expression profile in *Helicobacter pylori* clinical isolates. *Infect Immun* 2009, 77:3782-3790.

59. Yamaoka Y, Ojo O, Fujimoto S, Odenbreit S, Haas R, Gutierrez O, El-Zimaity HM, Reddy R, Arnqvist A, Graham DY: *Helicobacter pylori* outer membrane proteins and gastroduodenal disease. *Gut* 2006, 55:775-781.

60. Steffen Backert, Marguerite Clyne[2†] and Nicole Tegtmeyer[1.] Molecular mechanisms of gastric epithelial cell adhesion and injection of CagA by *Helicobacter pylori*. *Cell Communication and Signaling* 2011, 9:28 doi:10.1186/1478-811X-9-28

61. V. Chiozzi, G. Mazzini, A. Oldani, A. Sciullo, U. Ventura, M. Romano, P. Boquet, V. Ricci. Relationship Between Vac A Toxin And Ammonia

In Helicobacter Pylori-Induced Apoptosis In Human Gastric Epithelial Cells. *Journal of physiology and pharmacology* 2009, 60, 3, 23-30.

62. Galmiche A, Rassow J, Doye A, et al. The N-terminal 34 kDa fragment of Helicobacter pylori vacuolating cytotoxin targets mitochondria and induces cytocrome c release. *EMBO J.* 2000; 19: 6361-6370.

63. Yi-Chia Lee; Jyh-Ming Liou; Ming-Shiang Wu; Chun-Ying Wu; Jaw-Town Lin, 2008, Review: Eradication of Helicobacter pylori To Prevent Gastroduodenal Diseases: Hitting More Than One Bird With the Same Stone, *The AdvGastroenterol;* :111-120

64. YamaokaY., KatoM., and AsakaM. 2008. Geographic differences in gastric cancer incidence can be explained by differences between Helicobacter pylori strains. *Internal Medicine*, vol. 47, no. 12, pp. 1077–1083.

65. Sachs, George and Scott, David R., 2012, Helicobacter pylori: Eradication or Preservation, *F1000 Medicine Reports,* 4:7 (doi: 10.3410/M4-7). (http://f1000.com/reports/m/4/7).

66. Giorgio Floriana, Beatrice Principi Maria, De Francesco Vincenzo, Primary clarithromycin resistance to Helicobacter pylori: Is this the main reason for triple therapy failure? *World J Gastrointest Pathophysiology* 2013 August 15; 4(3): 43-46.

67. Wu, W., Yang, Y., and Sun, G. 2012. Recent insights into antibiotic resistance in Helicobacter pylori eradication. *Gastroenterology Research and Practice*. Volume (2012), Article ID 723183, http://dx.doi.org/10.1155/2012/723183.

68. Rimbara E, Fischbach LA, Graham DY. Optimal therapy for Helicobacter pylori infections. *Nat Rev Gastroenterol Hepatol.* 2011 Feb;8(2):79-88. doi: 10.1038/nrgastro.2010.210.

69. Frank I Tovey, Michael Hobsley, John Holton. Helicobacter pylori virulence factors in duodenal ulceration: A primary cause or a

secondary infection causing chronicity. *World J Gastroenterol* 2006 January 7; 12(1): 6-9.

70. Chey W, Wong B et al, *American College of Gastroenterology* Guideline on the Management of Helicobacter Pylori Infection, 2007, 102;1808-1825

71. V. De Francesco, F. Giorgio, C. Hassan et al., "Worldwide H. pylori antibiotic resistance: a systematic review," *Journal of Gastrointestinal and Liver Diseases*, vol. 19, no. 4, pp. 409–414, 2010

72. Gasparetto M., Pescarin M., and Guariso G.. Helicobacter pylori Eradication Therapy: Current Availabilities. *ISRN Gastroenterology Volume 2012* (2012), Article ID 186734, 8 pages http://dx.doi.org/10.5402/2012/186734.

73. Megraud F. H pylori antibiotic resistance: prevalence, importance, and advances in testing. *Gut* 2004; 53: 1374-1384.

74. Vincenzo De Francesco, Enzo Ierardi, Cesare Hassan, and Angelo Zullo. *Helicobacter pylori* therapy: Present and future. *World J Gastrointest Pharmacol Ther*. 2012 August 6; 3(4): 68–73. Published online 2012 August 6. doi: 10.4292/wjgpt.v3.i4.68. PMCID: PMC3437448

75. Bauer Bianca and Meyer F. Thomas. The Human Gastric Pathogen Helicobacter pylori and Its Association with Gastric Cancer and Ulcer Disease. *Ulcers*. Volume 2011 (2011), Article ID 340157, 23 pages http://dx.doi.org/10.1155/2011/340157.

76. Talley N. J., Ormand J. E., Frie C. A., and Zinsmeister A. R., "Stability of pH gradients in vivo across the stomach in Helicobacter pylori gastritis, dyspepsia, and health," *American Journal of Gastroenterology*, vol. 87, no. 5, pp. 590–594, 1992.

77. Kidd M. and Modlin I. M., "A century of Helicobacter pylori: paradigms lost-paradigms regained," *Digestion*, vol. 59, no. 1, pp. 1–15, 1998. View at Publisher · View at Google Scholar · View at Scopus

78. Warren J. R., "Unidentified curved bacilli on gastric epithelium in active chronic gastritis," *Lancet*, vol. 1, no. 8336, pp. 1273–1275, 1983.

79. Marshall B. J., Armstrong J. A., McGechie D. B., and. Glancy R. J, "Attempt to fulfil Koch's postulates for pyloric campylobacter," *Medical Journal of Australia*, vol. 142, no. 8, pp. 436–439, 1985. View at Scopus

80. Herbrink P, van Doorn LJ. Serological methods for diagnosis of Helicobacter pylori infection and monitoring of eradication therapy. *Eur J Clin Microbiol Infect Dis* 2000; 19: 164-173

81. Peters TM, Owen RJ, Slater E, Varea R, Teare EL, Saverymuttu S. Genetic diversity in the Helicobacter pylori cag pathogenicity island and effect on expression of anti-CagA serum antibody in UK patients with dyspepsia. *J Clin Pathol* 2001; 54: 219-223

82. Saribasak H, Salih BA, Yamaoka Y, Sander E. Analysis of Helicobacter pylori genotypes and correlation with clinical outcome in Turkey. *J Clin Microbiol* 2004; **42**: 1648-1651

83. Yang G, Hu F, Jia J. Relation between infection of CagA-positive *Helicobacter pylori* and upper gastrointestinal diseases. Zhonghua Yi Xue Za Zhi 2001; 81: 648–50.

84. Deguchi R., Igarashi M., Watanabe K. & A. Takagi. Analysis of the cag pathogenicity island and IS605 of Helicobacter pylori strains isolated from patients with gastric cancer in Japan. *Aliment Pharmacol Ther* 2004; 20 (Suppl. 1): 13–16.

85. Cover, T. L., Glupczynski Y., Lage A. P., Burette A., Tummuru M. K., Perez-Perez G. I., and. M. J. Blaser. 1995. Serologic detection of infection with *cagA⁺ Helicobacter pylori* strains. *J. Clin. Microbiol.* 33:1496-1500.

86. Enroth, H., O. Nyrén, and L. Engstrand. 1999. One stomach—one strain: does *Helicobacter pyori* strain variation influence disease outcome? *Dig. Dis. Sci.* 44:102-107.

87. Sicinschi LA, Correa P, Peek RM, Camargo MC, Delgado A, Piazuelo MB, Romero-Gallo J, Bravo LE, Schneider BG. Helicobacter pylori genotyping and sequencing using paraffin-embedded biopsies from residents of colombian areas with contrasting gastric cancer risks. *Helicobacter*. 2008;13:135–145.

88. Vega AE, Cortiñas TI, Puig ON, Silva HJ. Molecular characterization and susceptibility testing of Helicobacter pylori strains isolated in western Argentina. *Int J Infect Dis*. 2010;14 Suppl 3:e85–e92.

89. Suerbaum S, Josenhans C. Helicobacter pylori evolution and phenotypic diversification in a changing host. *Nat Rev Microbiol*. 2007;5:441–452.

90. Argent RH, Zhang Y, Atherton JC. Simple method for determination of the number of Helicobacter pylori CagA variable-region EPIYA tyrosine phosphorylation motifs by PCR. *J Clin Microbiol*. 2005;43:791–795.

91. Panayotopoulou EG, Sgouras DN, Papadakos K, Kalliaropoulos A, Papatheodoridis G, Mentis AF, Archimandritis AJ. Strategy to characterize the number and type of repeating EPIYA phosphorylation motifs in the carboxyl terminus of CagA protein in Helicobacter pylori clinical isolates. *J Clin Microbiol*. 2007;45:488–495.

92. Christina Nilsson, Anna Sillén, Lena Eriksson, Mona-Lisa Strand, Helena Enroth, Staffan Normark, Per Falk, and Lars Engstrand. Correlation between *cag* Pathogenicity Island Composition and *Helicobacter pylori*-Associated Gastroduodenal Disease. *Infect Immun*. 2003 November; 71(11): 6573–6581. doi: 10.1128/IAI.71.11.6573-6581.2003. PMCID: PMC219608.

93. Luciano Lobo Gatti[I,II], Roger de Lábio[I], Luiz Carlos da Silva[III], Marília de Arruda Cardoso Smith[II]; Spencer Luiz Marques Payao'. *cagA* positive *Helicobacter pylori* in Brazilian children related to chronic

gastritis *Braz J Infect* Dis vol.10 no.4 Salvador Aug. 2006. http://dx.doi.org/10.1590/S1413-86702006000400008.

94. Salama, N., K. Guillemin, T. K. McDaniel, G. Sherlock, L. Tompkins, and S. Falkow. 2000. A whole-genome microarray reveals genetic diversity among *Helicobacter pylori* strains. *Proc. Natl. Acad.* Sci. USA **97**:14668–14673.

95. Sozzi M, Tomasini ML, Vindigni C, Zanussi S, Tedeschi R, Basaglia G, et al. Heterogeneity of cag genotypes and clinical outcome of Helicobacter pylori infection. *J Lab Clin Med* 2005; 146:262–70.

96. Ikenoue T, Maeda S, Ogura K, Akanuma M, Mitsuno Y, Imai Y, et al. Determination of *Helicobacter pylori* virulence by simple gene analysis of the cag pathogenicity island. *Clin Diagn Lab Immunol* 2001; 8:181–6

97. Miehlke S, Kibler K, Kim JG, Figura N, Small SM, Graham DY, et al. Allelic variation in the cag A gene of Helicobacter pylori obtained from Korea compared to the United States. *Am J Gastroenterol* 1996; 91:1322–5

98. Valeska Portela Lima, Marcos Antonio Pereira de Lima, Marcia Valeria Pitombeira Ferreira a Marcos Aurelio Pessoa Barros, Sillvia Helena Barem Rabenhorst. The relationship between Helicobacter pylori genes cag E and vir B11 and gastric cancer. *International Journal of Infectious Diseases* 14 (2010) e613–e617.

99. Rocha G.A., Oliveira A.M., Queiroz D.M., Carvalho A.S., Nogueira A.M.. Immunoblot analysis of humoral immune response to *Helicobacter pylori* in children with and without duodenal ulcer. *J Clin Microbiol*, 38 (2000), pp. 1777–1781

100. Parsonnet J., Friedman G.D., Orentreich N., Vogelman H.. Risk for gastric cancer in people with CagA positive or CagA negative *Helicobacter pylori* infection. *Gut,* 40 (1997), pp. 297–301.

101. Hols O., Ulme A. J., Brad H., Fla H.-D., Rietsche E. T. Biochemistry and cell biology of bacterial endotoxins. *FEMS Immunol. Med. Microbiol.* 1996;16:83–104.

102. Rietschel, E. T., L. Brade, O. Holst, V. A. Kulshin, B. Lindner, A. P. Moran, U. F. Schade, U. Zähringer, and H. Brade. 1990. Molecular structure of bacterial endotoxin in relation to bioactivity, p. 15–32. *In* A. Nowotny, J. J. Spitzer, and E. J. Ziegler (ed.), *Endotoxin Research Series*, vol. 1. *Cellular and Molecular Aspects of Endotoxin Reactions.* Elsevier Science, Amsterdam, The Netherlands.

103. Rietschel, E. T., L. Brade, U. Schade, U. Seydel, U. Zähringer, O. Holst, H.-M. Kuhn, V. A. Kulschin, A. P. Moran, and H. Brade. 1991. Bacterial endotoxins: relationships between chemical structure and biological activity of the inner core-lipid A domain, p. 209–217. *In* E. Z. Ron and S. Rottem (ed.), *Microbial Surface Components and Toxins in Relation to Pathogenesis.* Plenum Press, New York, N.Y.

104. Goodwin C. S., Armstrong J. A., Chilvers T., Peters M., Collins M. D., Sly L., McConnel W., Harper W. E. S. Transfer of *Campylobacter pylori* and *Campylobacter mustelae* to *Helicobacter* gen. nov. as *Helicobacter pylori* comb. nov. and *Helicobacter mustelae* comb. nov., respectively. *Int. J. Syst. Bacteriol.* 1989; 39:397–405.

105. Lee A., Phillips M. W., O'Rourke J. L., Paster B. J., Dewhirst F. E., Fraser G. J., Fox J. G., Sly L. I., Romaniuk P. J., Trust T. J., Kouprach S. *Helicobacter muridarum* sp. nov., a microaerophilic helical bacterium with a novel ultrastructure isolated from the intestinal musosa of rodents. *Int. J. Syst. Bacteriol.* 1992;42:27–36.

106. Bode G., Mauch F., Ditschuneit H., Malfertheiner P. Identification of structures containing polyphosphate in *Helicobacter pylori. J. Gen. Microbiol.* 1993;139: 3029–3033.

107. Shahamat M, Mai U, Paszko-Kolva C, Yamamoto H, Colwell RR (1991) Evaluation of liquid media for growth of Helicobacter pylori. *J Clin Microbiol* 29:2835–2837

108. Jiang X, Doyle MP (2000) Growth supplements for Helicobacter pylori. *J Clin Microbiol* 38(5):1984–1987

109. Deshpande M, Calenoff E, Daniels L (1995) Rapid large-scale growth of Helicobacter pylori in flasks and fermentors. *Appl Environ Microbiol* 61(6):2431–2435.

110. Nedenskov P (1994) Nutritional requirements for growth of *Helicobacter pylori*. *Appl Environ Microbiol* 60(9):3450–3453

111. Reynolds DJ, Penn CW (1994) Characteristics of *Helicobacter pylori* growth in a defined medium and determination of its amino acid requirements. *Microbiology* 140:2649–2656

112. Morshed MG, Karita M, Konishi H, Okita K, Nakazawa T (1994). Growth medium containing cyclodextrin and low concentration of horse serum for cultivation of Helicobacter pylori. *Microbiol Immunol* 38(11):897–900.

113. Kitsos CM, Stadtländer CT (1998) *Helicobacter pylori* in liquid culture: evaluation of growth rates and ultrastructure. *Curr Microbiol* 37(2):88–93. doi:10.1007/s002849900344

114. Vega AE, Cortiñas TI, Mattana CM, Silva HJ, Puig De Centorbi O (2003) Growth of *Helicobacter pylori* in medium supplemented with cyanobacterial extract. *J Clin Microbiol* 41(12):5384–5388. doi:10.1128/JCM.41.12.5384-5388.2003.

115. Jay V. Solnick and Peter Vandamme. Helicobacter pylori, Physiology and Genetics. Edited by Harry LT Mobley, George L Mendz, and Stuart L Hazell. Washington (DC): ASM Press; 2001. ISBN-10: 1-55581-213-9

116. Goodwin C. S., McCulloch R. K., Armstrong J. A., Wee S. H. Unusual cellular fatty acids and distinctive ultrastructure in a new spiral

bacterium (*Campylobacter pyloridis*) from the human gastric mucosa. *J. Med. Microbiol.* 1985;19:257–267. [PubMed].

117. Jones D. M., Curry A., Fox A. J. An ultrastructural study of the gastric campylobacter-like organism "*Campylobacter pyloridis. J. Gen. Microbiol.* 1985; 131: 2335–2341.

118. Worku M. L., Sidebotham R. L., Walker M. M., Keshavarz T., Karim Q. N. The relationship between *Helicobacter pylori* motility, morphology and phase of growth: implications for gastric colonization and pathology. *Microbiology.* 1999; 145: 2803–2811.

119. Eaton K. A., Morgan D. R., Krakowka S. Motility as a factor in the colonization of gnotobiotic piglets by *Helicobacter pylori. J. Med. Microbiol.* 1992; 37:123–127. [PubMed].

120. Depamphilis M. L., Adler J. Attachment of flagellar basal bodies to the cell envelope: specific attachment to the outer, lipopolysaccharide membrane and the cytoplasmic membrane. *J. Bacteriol.* 1971;105:396–407. [PMC free article] [PubMed].

121. Benaissa M., Babin P., Quellard N., Pezennec L., Cenatiempo Y., Fauchere J. L. Changes in *Helicobacter pylori* ultrastructure and antigens during conversion from the bacillary to the coccoid form. *Infect. Immun.* 1996;64:2331–2335.

122. Kusters J. G., Gerrits M. M., Vanstrijp J., Vandenbrouckegrauls C. Coccoid forms of *Helicobacter pylori* are the morphologic manifestation of cell death. *Infect. Immun.* 1997;65:3672–3679. [PMC free article] [PubMed]

123. Aspinall G. O., Monteiro M. A., Pang H., Walsh E. J., Moran A. P. Lipopolysaccharide of the *Helicobacter pylori* type strain NCTC 11637 (ATCC 43504): structure of the O antigen chain and core oligosaccharide regions. *Biochemistry.* 1996;35:2489–2497.

124. Monteiro M. A., Chan K. H., Rasko D. A., Taylor D. E., Zheng P. Y., Appelmelk B. J., Wirth H. P., Yang M., Blaser M. J., Hynes S. O.,

Moran A. P., Perry M. B. Simultaneous expression of type 1 and type 2 Lewis blood group antigens by *Helicobacter pylori* lipopolysaccharides. Molecular mimicry between *H. pylori* lipopolysaccharides and human gastric epithelial cell surface glycoforms. *J. Biol.* Chem. 1998;273:11533–11543.

125. Appelmelk B. J., Shiberu B., Trinks C., Tapsi N., Zheng P. Y., Verboom T., Maaskant J., Hokke C. H., Schiphorst W. E., Blanchard D., Simoons-Smit I. M., van den Eijnden D. H., Vandenbroucke-Grauls C. M. Phase variation in *Helicobacter pylori* lipopolysaccharide. *Infect. Immun.* 1998; 66:70–76.

126. Mónica Oleastro 1 and Armelle Ménard 2,3,* The Role of Helicobacter pylori Outer Membrane Proteins in Adherence and Pathogenesis *Biology* 2013, *2*, 1110-1134; doi:10.3390/biology2031110.

127. González, C.; Megraud, F.; Buissonniere, A.; Lujan Barroso, L.; Agudo, A.; Duell, E.J.; Boutron-Ruault, M.C.; Clavel-Chapelon, F.; Palli, D.; Krogh, V.; *et al. Helicobacter pylori* infection assessed by ELISA and by immunoblot and noncardia gastric cancer risk in a prospective study: The Eurgast-EPIC project. *Ann. Oncol.* 2012, *23*, 1320–1324.

128. Banic, M.; Franceschi, F.; Babic, Z.; Gasbarrini, A. Extragastric manifestations of *Helicobacter pylori* infection. *Helicobacter* 2012, *17*, 49–55.

129. Fukase, K.; Kato, M.; Kikuchi, S.; Inoue, K.; Uemura, N.; Okamoto, S.; Terao, S.; Amagai, K.; Hayashi, S.; Asaka, M.; The Japan Gast Study Group. Effect of eradication of *Helicobacter pylori* on incidence of metachronous gastric carcinoma after endoscopic resection of early gastric cancer: An open-label, randomised controlled trial. *Lancet* 2008, *372*, 392–397.

130. Muotiala, A.; Helander, I.M.; Pyhala, L.; Kosunen, T.U.; Moran, A.P. Low biological activity of *Helicobacter pylori* lipopolysaccharide. *Infect. Immun.* 1992, *60*, 1714–1716.

131. Monteiro, M.A.; Appelmelk, B.J.; Rasko, D.A.; Moran, A.P.; Hynes, S.O.; MacLean, L.L.; Chan, K.H.; Michael, F.S.; Logan, S.M.; O'Rourke, J.; *et al.* Lipopolysaccharide structures of *Helicobacter pylori* genomic strains 26695 and J99, mouse model *H-pylori* Sydney strain, *H-pylori* P466 carrying sialyl Lewis X, and *H-pylori* UA915 expressing Lewis B—Classification of *H-pylori* lipopolysaccharides into glycotype families. *Eur. J. Biochem.* 2000, *267*, 305–320.

132. Edwards, N.J.; Monteiro, M.A.; Faller, G.; Walsh, E.J.; Moran, A.P.; Roberts, I.S.; High, N.J.,Lewis X structures in the O antigen side-chain promote adhesion of *Helicobacter pylori* to the gastric epithelium. *Mol. Microbiol.* 2000, *35*, 1530–1539.

133. Monteiro, M.A.; Chan, K.H.N.; Rasko, D.A.; Taylor, D.E.; Zheng, P.Y.; Appelmelk, B.J.; Wirth, H.P.; Yang, M.; Blaser, M.J.; Hynes, S.O.; *et al.* Simultaneous expression of type 1 and type 2 Lewis blood group antigens by *Helicobacter pylori* lipopolysaccharides. *J. Biol. Chem.* 1998, *273*, 11533–11543.

134. Osaki, T.; Yamaguchi, H.; Taguchi, H.; Fukuda, M.; Kawakami, H.; Hirano, H.; Watanabe, S.; Takagi, A.; Kamiya, S. Establishment and characterisation of a monoclonal antibody to inhibit adhesion of *Helicobacter pylori* to gastric epithelial cells. *J. Med. Microbiol.* 1998, *47*, 505–512.

135. Fowler, M.; Thomas, R.J.; Atherton, J.; Roberts, I.S.; High, N.J. Galectin-3 binds to *Helicobacter pylori* O-antigen: It is upregulated and rapidly secreted by gastric epithelial cells in response to *H. pylori* adhesion. *Cell. Microbiol.* **2006**, *8*, 44–54.

136. Odenbreit, S.; Faller, G.; Haas, R. Role of the AlpAB proteins and lipopolysaccharide in adhesion of *Helicobacter pylori* to human gastric tissue. *Int. Med. Microbiol.* **2002**, *292*, 247–256

137. Mahdavi, J.; Boren, T.; Vandenbroucke Grauls, C.; Appelmelk, B.J. Limited role of lipopolysaccharide lewis antigens in adherence of *Helicobacter pylori* to the human gastric epithelium. *Infect. Immun.* 2003, *71*, 2876–2880.

138. Alm, R.A.; Bina, J.; Andrews, B.M.; Doig, P.; Hancock, R.E.W.; Trust, T.J. Comparative genomics of *Helicobacter pylori*: Analysis of the outer membrane protein families. *Infect. Immun.* 2000, *68*, 4155–4168.

139. Gernot Posselt, Steffen Backert and Silja Wessler. The functional interplay of *Helicobacter pylori* factors with gastric epithelial cells induces a multi-step process in pathogenesis.

140. Smith MF Jr, Mitchell A, Li G, Ding S, Fitzmaurice AM, Ryan K, Crowe S, Goldberg JB: Toll-like receptor (TLR) 2 and TLR5, but not TLR4, are required for *Helicobacter pylori*-induced NF-kappa B activation and chemokine expression by epithelial cells. *J Biol Chem* 2003, 278:32552-32560

141. Ishijima N, Suzuki M, Ashida H, Ichikawa Y, Kanegae Y, Saito I, Borén T, Haas R, Sasakawa C, Mimuro H: BabA-mediated adherence is a potentiator of the h*elicobacter pylori* type IV secretion system activity. *J Biol Chem* 2011, 286:25256-25264.

142. Rad R, Gerhard M, Lang R, Schoniger M, Rosch T, Schepp W, Becker I, Wagner H, Prinz C: The *Helicobacter pylori* blood group antigen-binding adhesin facilitates bacterial colonization and augments a nonspecific immune response. *J Immunol* 2002, 168:3033-3041

143. Gerhard M, Lehn N, Neumayer N, Boren T, Rad R, Schepp W, Miehlke S, Classen M, Prinz C: Clinical relevance of the *Helicobacter*

pylori gene for blood-group antigen-binding adhesin. *Proc Natl Acad Sci USA* 1999, 96:12778-12783

144. Lee SK, Stack A, Katzowitsch E, Aizawa SI, Suerbaum S, Josenhans C: *Helicobacter pylori* flagellins have very low intrinsic activity to stimulate human gastric epithelial cells via TLR5. *Microbes Infect* 2003, 5:1345-1356.

145. Andersen-Nissen E, Smith KD, Strobe KL, Barrett SL, Cookson BT, Logan SM, Aderem A: Evasion of toll-like receptor 5 by flagellated bacteria. *Proc Natl Acad Sci USA* 2005, 102:9247-9252.

146. Morris, A.; Nicholson, G.; Zwi, J.; Vanderwee, M. *Campylobacter pylori* infection in Meckel's diverticula containing gastric mucosa. *Gut* 1989, *30*, 1233–1235.

147. Kestemberg, A.; Mariño, G.; de Lima, E.; Garcia, F.; Carrascal, E.; Arredondo, J.L. Gastric heterotopic mucosa in the rectum with *Helicobacter pylori*-like organisms: A rare cause of rectal bleeding. *Int. J. Colorectal Dis.* 1993, *8*, 9–12.

148. Genta, R.M.; Gurer, I.E.; Graham, D.Y.; Krishnan, B.; Segura, A.M.; Gutierrez, O.; Kim, J.G.; Burchette, J.L., Jr. Adherence of *Helicobacter pylori* to areas of incomplete intestinal metaplasia in the gastric mucosa. *Gastroenterology* 1996, *111*, 1206–1211.

149. Oleastro, M.; Cordeiro, R.; Ferrand, J.; Nunes, B.; Lehours, P.; Carvalho-Oliveira, I.; Mendes, A.L.; Monteiro, L.; Mégraud, F.; Ménard, A. Evaluation of the clinical significance of *hom*B, a novel candidate marker of *Helicobacter pylori* strains associated with peptic ulcer disease. *J. Infect.Dis.* 2008, *198*, 1379–1387.

150. Dixon MF. Pathophysiology of Helicobacter pylori infection. Scandinavian Journal of Gastroenterology. Supplement 1994; 201: 7-10.

151. Sobala GM, Crabtree JE, Dixon MF, Schorah CJ, Taylor JD, Rathbone BJ, Heatly RV, Axon ATR. Acute Helicobacter pylori

infection: clinical features, local and systemic immune response, gastric mucosal histology, and gastric juice ascorbic acid concentrations. Gut 1991; 32: 1415-1418.

152. Crabtree JE, Taylor JD, Wyatt JL, Heatly RV, Shallcross TM, Tompkins DS, Rathbone BJ. Mucosal IgA recognition of Helicobacter pylori 120kDa protein, peptic ulceration and gastric pathology. Lancet 1991; 338: 332-335.

153. Rathobone BJ, Wyatt JI, Worsley BW, Shires SE, Trejdosiewicz LK, Heatley RV, Losowsky MS. Systemic and local antibody responses to gastric Campylobacter pyloridis in non-ulcer dyspepsia. Gut 1986; 27: 642-647.

154. McColl KEL, El Omar E, Gillen D. Interactions between *H. pylori* infection, gastric acid secretion and anti-secretory therapy. British Medical Bulletin 1998; 54: 121-138.

155. Dixon MF. Pathology of gastritis and peptic ulceration. In mobley HLT, Mendz GL and Hazell SL., ed. *Helicobacter pylori*: Physiology and genetics. Washington DC: ASM Press, 2001; 459-470.

156. Egan B, Holmes K, Humphrey J, Helicobacter pylori gastritis, the unifying concept for gastric diseases, Helicobacter 2007 (12); 39-44

157. Weck M, Gao L, Brenner H, Helicobacter pylori infection and chronic atrophic gastritis: associations according to severity of disease, Epidemiology 2009, 20(4), 569-74

158. Sleisenger and Fordtran's Gastrointestinal and Liver Disease, 9th edition, 2010, chapter 13

159. Talley NJ, Vakil NB, Moayyedi P: American Gastroenterological Association technical review on the evaluation of dyspepsia. *Gastroenterology* 2005; 129:1756-80.

160. Atherton JC. The pathogenesis of *Helicobacter pylori* – induced gastro-duodenal diseases. Annual Review of Pathology 2006; 1: 63-96.

161. Walsh JH, Peterson WL. The treatment of *Helicobacter pylori* infection in the management of peptic ulcer disease. New England Journal of Medicine 1995; 333: 984-991.

162. Forbes GM, Glaser ME, Cullen DJ, Warren JR, Christiansen KJ, B.J.M, Collins BJ. Duodenal ulcer treated with Helicobacter pylori eradication: seven year follow-up. Lancet 1994; 343: 258-260.

163. Graham DY, Lew GM, Klein PD, D.G.E., Evans DJJ, Saeed ZA, Malaty HM. Effect of treatment of *Helicobacter pylori* infection on the long-term recurrence of gastric or duodenal ulcer. A randomized, controlled study. Annals of Internal Medicine 1992; 116: 705-708.

164. Hentschel E, Brandstatter G, Dragosics B, Hirschl AM, Nemec H, Schutze K, Taufer M, Wurzer H. Effect of ranitidine and amoxicillin plus metronidazole on eradication of *Helicobacter pylori* and the recurrence of duodenal ulcer. New England Journal of Medicine 1993; 328: 308-312.

165. Triantafillidis J.K, Triantafillidis H., Extragastric manifestations of H. pylori infection: a critical reappraisal, Annals of Gastroenterology 2006, 19 (2), 110-115

166. El-Omar EM, Penman ID, Ardill JES, Chittajallu RS, Howie C, McColl KEL. *Helicobacter pylori* infection and abnormalities of acid secretion in patients with duodenal ulcer disease. Gastroenterology 1995; 109: 681-691.

167. El-Omar EM, Oien K, elNujumi A, GillenD, Wirz A, Dahill S, Williams C, Ardill JES, McColl KEL. Helicobacter pylori infection and chronic gastric acid hyposecretion. Gastroenterology, 1997; 113: 15-24.

168. Khulusi S, Badve S, Patel P, Lloyd R, Marrero JM, Finlayson C, Mendall MA, Northfield TC. Pathogenesis of gastric metaplasia of the human duodenum: Role of Helicobacter pylori, gastric acid, and ulceration. Gastroenterology 1996. 110: 452-458.

169. Peek, R. M., Jr. & Blaser, M. J. (2002). *Helicobacter pylori* and gastrointestinal tract adenocarcinomas. *Nat Rev Cancer* **2**, 28-37.

170. Prinz, C., Schoniger, M., Rad, R. & other authors (2001). Key importance of the *Helicobacter pylori* adherence factor blood group antigen binding adhesin during chronic gastric inflammation. *Cancer Res* 61, 1903-1909.

171. Gerhard, M., Lehn, N., Neumayer, N., Borén, T., Rad, R., Schepp, W., Miehlke, S., Classen, M. & Prinz, C. (1999). Clinical relevance of the *Helicobacter pylori* gene for blood-group antigen-binding adhesin. *Proc Natl Acad Sci U S A* 96, 12778-12783.

172. Xiang, Z., Censini, S., Bayeli, P. F., Telford, J. L., Figura, N., Rappuoli, R. & Covacci, A. (1995). Analysis of expression of CagA and VacA virulence factors in 43 strains of *Helicobacter pylori* reveals that clinical isolates can be divided into two major types and that CagA is not necessary for expression of the vacuolating cytotoxin. *Infect Immun* 63, 94-98.

173. El-Omar E.M., Carrington M., Chow W.H., McColl K.E., Bream J.H., Young H.A. et al. (2000) Interleukin-1 polymorphisms associated with increased risk of gastric cancer. *Nature* 404:398–402. [PubMed].

174. El-Omar E.M., Rabkin C.S., Gammon M.D., Vaughan T.L., Risch H.A., Schoenberg J.B. et al. (2003) Increased risk of noncardia gastric cancer associated with proinflammatory cytokine gene polymorphisms. *Gastroenterology* 124:1193–1201. [PubMed].

175. Parkin DM, Bray F, Ferlay J, Pisani P. Global cancer statistics. 2005. *CA Cancer J. Clin.* 2005; 55: 74–108.

176. Huang JQ, Zheng GF, Sumanac K *et al.* Meta-analysis of the relationship between *caga* seropositivity and gastric cancer. *Gastroenterology* 2003; 125: 1636–44.

177. El-Omar EM, Oien K, El Nujumi A *et al.* *Helicobacter pylori* infection and chronic gastric acid hyposecretion. *Gastroenterology* 1997; 113: 15–24.

178. Suerbaum S, Michetti P. Helicobacter pylori infection. *N. Engl. J. Med.* 2002; 347: 1175–86.

179. Correa P, Piazuelo MB, Camargo MC. The future of gastric cancer prevention. *Gastric Cancer.* 2004; **7**: 9–16.

180. Chien-Yu Lu, Chao-Hung Kuo, Yi-Ching Lo, Hung-Yi Chuang, Yuan-Chieh Yang, I-Chen Wu, Fang-Jong Yu, Yi-Chen Lee, 2005, *The best method of detecting prior Helicobacter pylori infection,* World J Gastroenterol2005;11(36):5672-5676

181. Chan Gyoo Kim; Il Ju Choi; Jong Yeul Lee; Soo-Jeong Cho; Byung-Ho Nam; Myeong-Cherl Kook; Eun Kyung Hong, 2009, *Biopsy Site for Detecting Helicobacter Pylori Infection in Patients with Gastric Cancer,* J Gastroenterol Hepatol, 469-474

182. Ilie Madalina, Dascalu Luminita, Chifiriuc Carmen, Popa Marcela, Constantinescu Gabriel, Tanasescu Coman, Baltac Alina. Correlation of anti- *Helicobacter pylori* cagA IgG antibodies with resistance to first line treatment, bleeding gastroduodenal ulcers and gastric cancer. Romanian Archives of Microbiology and Immunology. 2011. 70 (3): 101-104.

183. Malfertheiner Peter, M.D.; Sipponen Pentti, M.D.; Naumann Michael, Ph.D.; Paul Moayyedi.; Francis Mégraud; 2005; *Helicobacter pylori Eradication Has the Potential to Prevent Gastric Cancer: A State-of-the-Art Critique*; The American Journal of Gastroenterology, 2100-2115

184. Ilie Mădălina, Popa Marcela, Chifiriuc Mariana Carmen, Baltac Alina, Constantinescu Gabriel, Tănăsescu Coman, 2011, *Helicobacter pylori cultivation from gastric biopsies and susceptibility to antibiotics used in*

empirical therapy, Romanian Archives of Microbiology and Immunology (2:60-64)

185. Sachs George, Scott R. David. *Helicobacter pylori*: Eradication or Preservation. F1000 Med Rep. 2012; 4: 7. Published online 2012 April 2. doi: 10.3410/M4-7

186. Malfertheiner P., Megraud F., O'Morain C. et al., "Current concepts in the management of *Helicobacter pylori* infection: the Maastricht III Consensus Report," *Gut*, vol. 56, no. 6, pp. 772–781, 2007.

187. Basu P. P., Rayapudi K., Pacana T., Shah N. J., N. Krishnaswamy, and M. Flynn, "A randomized study comparing levofloxacin, omeprazole, nitazoxanide, and doxycycline versus triple therapy for the eradication of *Helicobacter pylori*," *The American Journal of Gastroenterology*, vol. 106, no. 11, pp. 1970–1975, 2011.

188. Hsu P. I., Wu D. C., Chen A. et al., "Quadruple rescue therapy for *Helicobacter pylori* infection after two treatment failures, *European Journal of Clinical Investigation*, vol. 38, no. 6, pp. 404–409, 2008.

189. Ueki N., Miyake K, Kusunoki M., Shindo T, Kawagoe T, Futagami S. et al. (2009)Impact of quadruple regimen of clarithromycin added to metronidazole-containing triple therapy against Helicobacter pylori infection following clarithromycin-containing triple-therapy failure. *Helicobacter* 14:91–99.

190. Murakami K, Okimoto T, Kodama M., Sato R., Watanabe K., Fujioka T. (2008) Evaluation of three different proton pump inhibitors with amoxicillin and metronidazole in retreatment for Helicobacter pylo ri infection. *J Clin Gastroenterol* 42:139–142.

191. Murakami K, Okimoto T, Kodama M., Sato R., Miyajima H., Ono M. et al. (2006)Comparison of amoxicillin-metronidazole plus famotidine or lansoprazole for amoxicillin-clarithromycin-proton pump inhibitor treatment failures for Helicobacter pylori infection. *Helicobacter* 11:436–440.

192. Shirai N., Sugimoto M., Kodaira C, Nishino M., Ikuma M., Kajimura M. et al. (2007) Dual therapy with high doses of rabeprazole and amoxicillin versus triple therapy with rabeprazole, amoxicillin, and metronidazole as a rescue regimen for *Helicobacter pylori* infection after the standard triple therapy. *Eur J Clin Pharmacol* 63:743–749.

193. Matsuhisa T, Kawai T, Masaoka T, Suzuki H., Ito M., Kawamura Y. et al. (2006) Efficacy of metronidazole as second-line drug for the treatment of Helicobacter pylori infection in the Japanese population: a multicenter study in the Tokyo metropolitan area. *Helicobacter* 11:152–158.

194. Nagahara A., Miwa H., Kawabe M., Kurosawa A., Asaoka D., Hojo M. et al. (2004) Second-line treatment for Helicobacter pylori infection in Japan: proton pump inhibitor-based amoxicillin and metronidazole regimen. *J Gastroenterol* 39:1051–1055.

195. Shimoyama T., Fukuda S., Mikami T., Fukushi M., Munakata A.(2004)Efficacy of metronidazole for the treatment of clarithromycin-resistant Helicobacter pylori infection in a Japanese population. *J Gastroenterol* 39:927–930.

196. Isomoto H., Inoue K., Furusu H., Enjoji A., Fujimoto C., Yamakawa M. et al. (2003)High-dose rabeprazole-amoxicillin versus rabeprazole-amoxicil-lin-metronidazole as second-line treatment after failure of the Japanese standard regimen for Helicobacter pylori infection. *Aliment Pharmacol Ther* 18:101–107.

197. Miwa H., Nagahara A., Kurosawa A., Ohkusa T, Ohkura R., Hojo M. et al. (2003)Is antimicrobial susceptibility testing necessary before second-line treatment for Helicobacter pylori infection? *Aliment Pharmacol Ther* 17:1545–1551.

198. Malfertheiner P., Megraud F., O'Morain C, Bazzoli F., El-Omar E., Graham D. et al. (2007) Current Concepts in the Management of

Helicobacter pylori Infection: The Maastricht III Consensus Report. Gut 56:772–781.

199. Gisbert J.P., Calvet X., Gomollon F., Sainz R. (2000) [Treatment for the eradication of Helicobacter pylori. Recommendations of the Spanish Consensus Conference].*Med Clin* (Barc) 114:185–195.

200. Lam S.K, Talley N.J.(1998) Report of the 1997 Asia Pacific Consensus Conference on the Management of Helicobacter pylori Infection. *J Gastroenterol Hepatol* 13:1–12.

201. Rispo A., Di Girolamo E., Cozzolino A., Bozzi R., Morante A., Pasquale L.(2007)Levofloxacin in first-line treatment of Helicobacter pylori infection. *Helicobacter* 12:364–365.

202. Gisbert J.P., Fernandez-Bermejo M., Molina-Infante J., Perez-Gallardo B., Prieto-Bermejo A.B., Mateos-Rodriguez J.M. et al. (2007). First-line triple therapy with levofloxacin for Helicobacter pylori eradication. *Aliment Pharmacol Ther* 26:495–500.

203. Antos D., Schneider-Brachert W., Bastlein E., Hanel C, Haferland C, Buchner M. et al. (2006)7-day triple therapy of Helicobacter pylori infection with levofloxacin, amoxicillin, and high-dose esomeprazole in patients with known antimicrobial sensitivity. *Helicobacter* 11:39–45.

204. Lee J.H., Hong S.P., Kwon C.I., Phyun L.H., Lee B.S., Song H.U. et al. (2006a)[The efficacy of levofloxacin based triple therapy for Helicobacter pylori eradication]. *Korean J Gastroenterol* 48:19–24.

205. Marzio L., Coraggio D., Capodicasa S., Grossi L., Cappello G.(2006)Role of the preliminary susceptibility testing for initial and after failed therapy of Helicobacter pylori infection with levofloxacin, amoxi-cillin, and esomeprazole. *Helicobacter* 11:237–242.

206. Di Caro S., Assunta Zocco M., Cremonini F., Candelli M., Nista E.C., Bartolozzi F. et al. (2002)Levofloxacin based regimens for the eradication of Helicobacter pylori. *Eur J Gastroenterol Hepatol* 14:1309–1312.

207. Cammarota G., Cianci R., Cannizzaro O., Cuoco L., Pirozzi G., Gasbarrini A. et al. (2000)Efficacy of two one-week rabeprazole/levofloxacin-based triple therapies for Helicobacter pylori infection. *Aliment Pharmacol Ther* 14:1339–1343.

208. Liou J. M., Lin J. T., Chang C. Y. et al., "Levofloxacin-based and clarithromycin-based triple therapies as first-line and secondline treatments for *Helicobacter pylori* infection: a randomized comparative trial with crossover design," *Gut*, vol. 59, no. 5, pp. 572–578, 2010

209. On SLW. Taxonomy of *Campylobacter*, *Arcobacter*, *Helicobacter* and related bacteria: current status, future prospects and immediate concerns. *Journal of Applied Microbiology* 2001; 90: 1S-15S.

210. Schreiber S., Konradt M, Groll C, Scheid P, Hanauer G, Werling HO, Josenhans C, Suerbaum S. The spatial orientation of Helicobacter pylori in the gastric mucus. Proceedings of the National Academy of Sciences of the United States of America 2004; 101: 5024-5029.

211. Dubois A, Boren T. Helicobacter pylori is invasive and it may be a facultative intracellular organism. *Cellular Microbiology* 2007; 9: 1108-1116.

212. Malfertheiner P, Francis Megraud, Colm A O'Morain, John Atherton, Anthony T R Axon, Franco Bazzoli, Gian Franco Gensini, Javier P Gisbert, David Y Graham,Theodore Rokkas, Emad M El-Omar,Ernst J Kuipers- The European *H.* Study Group (EHSG)- *Management of H. pylori infection the Maastricht IV/ Florence Consensus Report*,2012

213. Malfertheiner P, Megraud F, O'Morain C, et al. Current concepts in the management of *H. pylori* infection: *the Maastricht III Consensus Report. Gut*; 56:772, *2007*

214. Mégraud F, Lehours P. *H. pylori* detection and antimicrobial susceptibility testing. *Clin Microbiol Rev*; 20:280, 2007

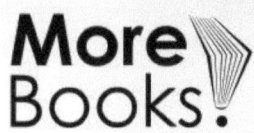
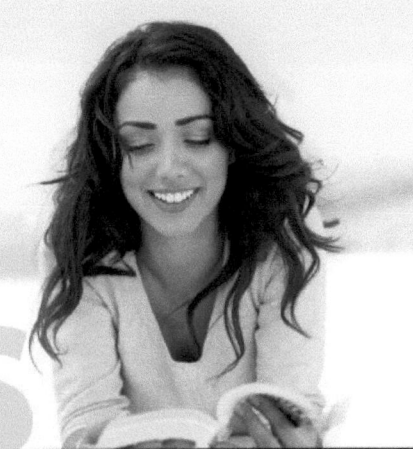

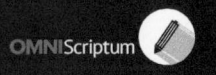

Printed by Books on Demand GmbH, Norderstedt / Germany

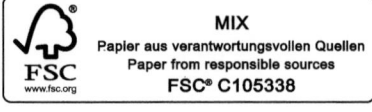

Printed by Books on Demand GmbH, Norderstedt / Germany